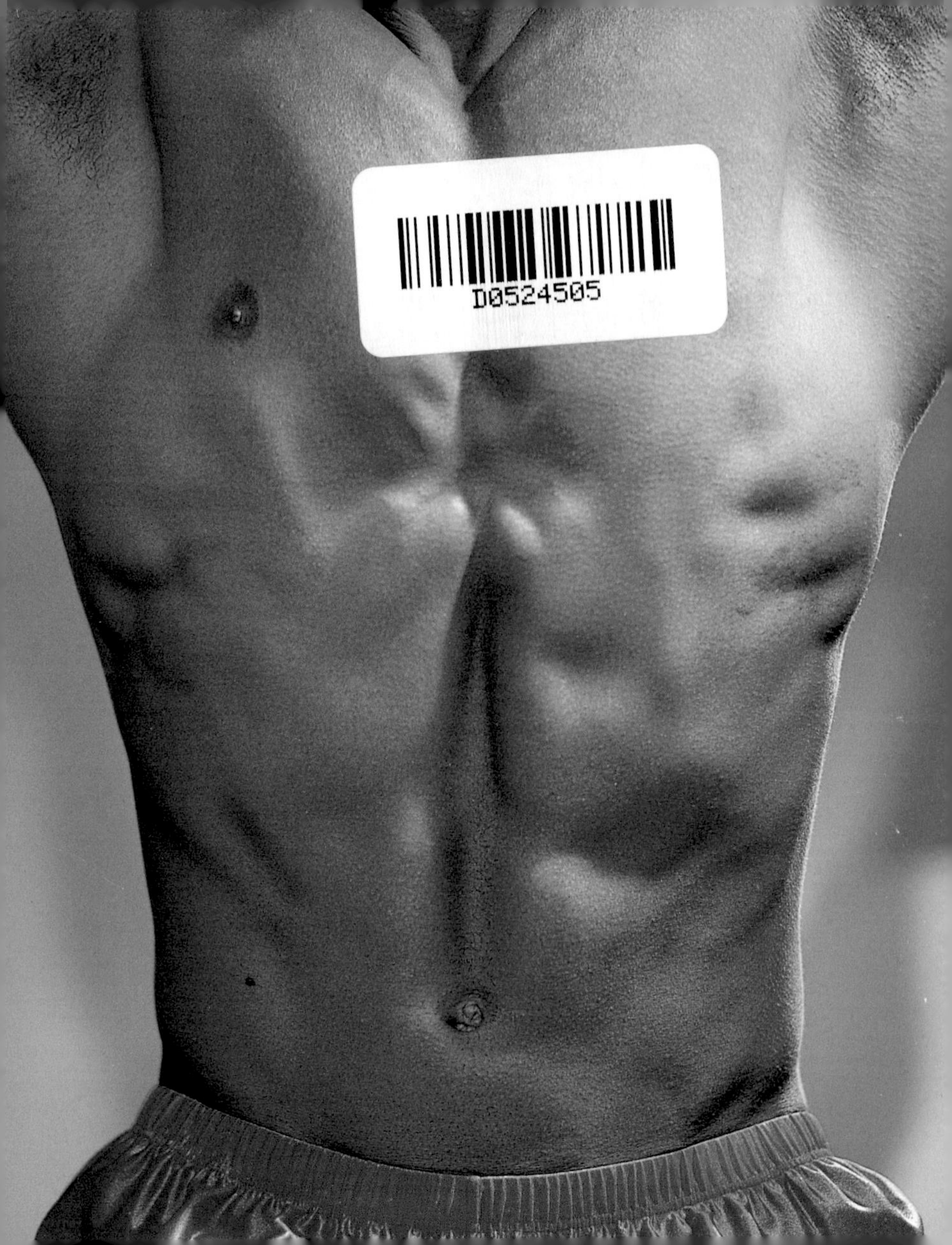

D0524505

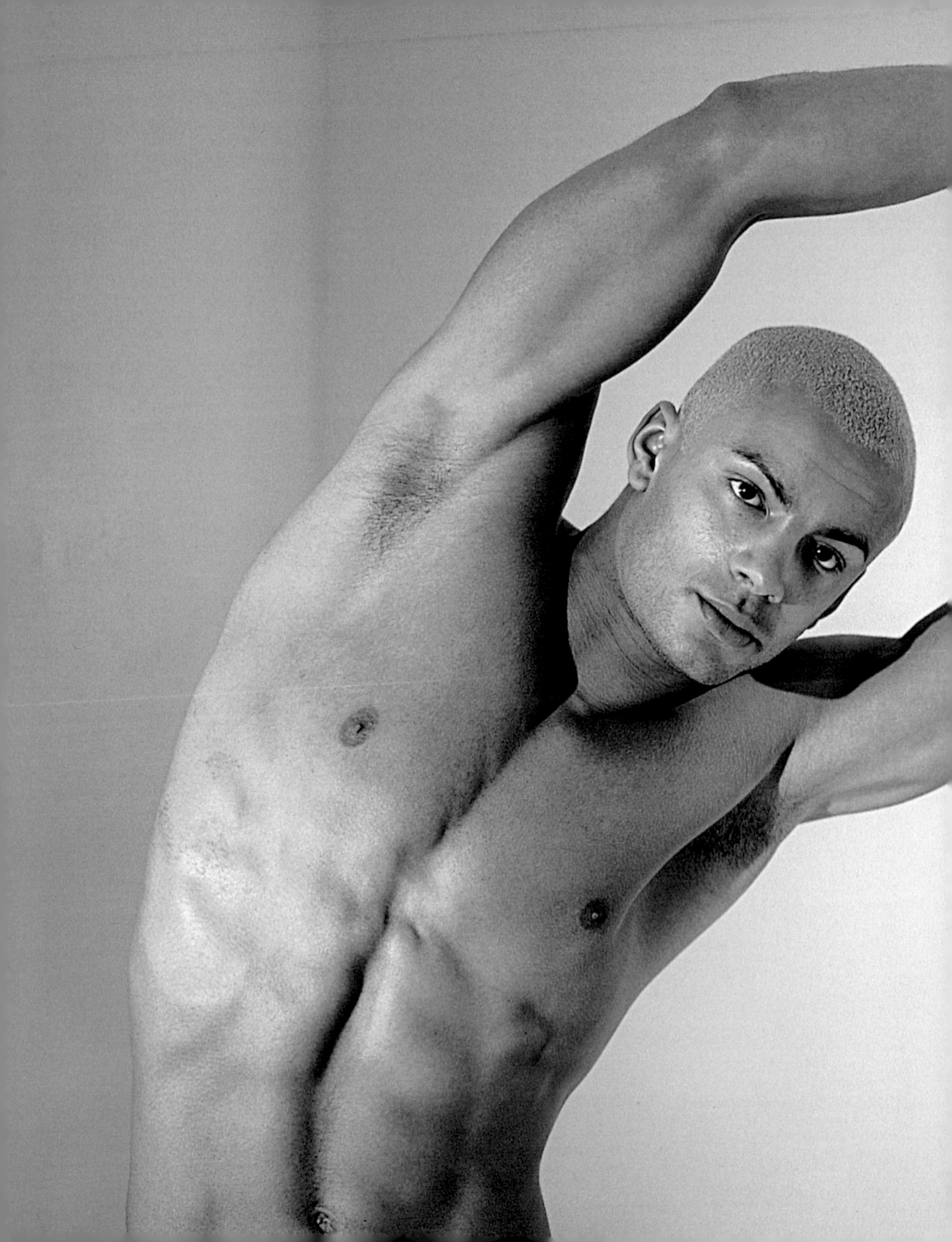

Matt Roberts

six-pack abs

A Dorling Kindersley Book

LONDON, NEW YORK, MUNICH,
MELBOURNE, and DELHI

This book is for my team at Jermyn Street

Editors Michael Fullalove, Anna Fischel
Project Art Editors Paul Reid, Darren Bland for Cobaltid
Managing Editor Gillian Roberts
Category Publisher Mary-Clare Jerram
Art Director Tracy Killick
DTP Designer Sonia Charbonnier
Production Controller Louise Daly
Photographer Russell Sadur

First published in Great Britain in 2003
by Dorling Kindersley Limited
80 Strand, London WC2R 0RL
A Penguin Company

Copyright © 2003 Dorling Kindersley Limited, London
Text Copyright © 2003 Matt Roberts Personal Training

4 6 8 10 9 7 5 3

Always consult your doctor before starting a fitness and/or nutrition programme if you have any health concerns.

All rights reserved. No part of this publication may be reproduced, stored in a retrieval system, or transmitted in any form or by any means, electronic, mechanical, photocopying or otherwise, without the prior written permission of the copyright owners.

A CIP catalogue record for this book is available from The British Library

ISBN 0 7513 4876 7

Colour reproduced by GRB, Italy

Printed and bound by Printer Trento, Italy

See our complete catalogue at www.dk.com

contents

foreword

about the book

If ever there was an international benchmark of how fit you are, it's got to be whether or not you have a six-pack – a set of stomach muscles so chiselled and toned they resemble an old-fashioned washboard. Six-packs rank high on the wishlists of most of the guys who come to my gym. They're the subject of many of the questions journalists put to me. And – on a purely personal level – they're where I get a testing prod the moment people find out I'm a trainer.

And yet, so much that's written about six-packs is pretty poor-quality stuff. Well, luckily, that's all about to change. Whether you're a newcomer to the whole business or are pegging away doing rep after rep day in, day out and feeling a bit disappointed with the results, this is the book for you.

Perfect abs don't come easily, I grant you. You can do as many sit-ups as you like, but if everything else you're doing is not quite right, the chances are high that your newly toned muscles will remain hidden under a layer of fat. The secret to six-pack sculpting lies in a combination of three things. Firstly, you need a progressive programme of intensive exercises, and the three workouts I've put together for you

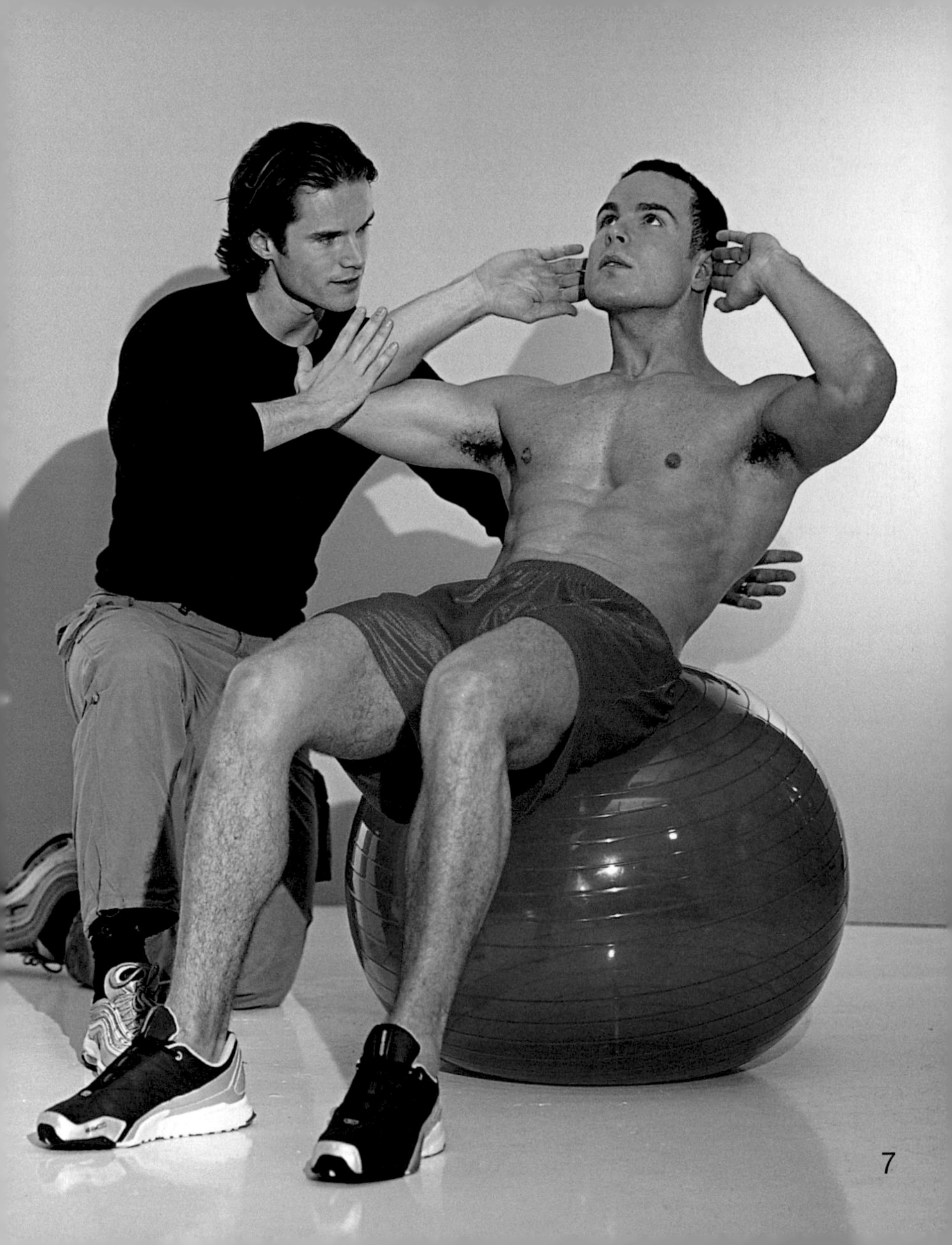

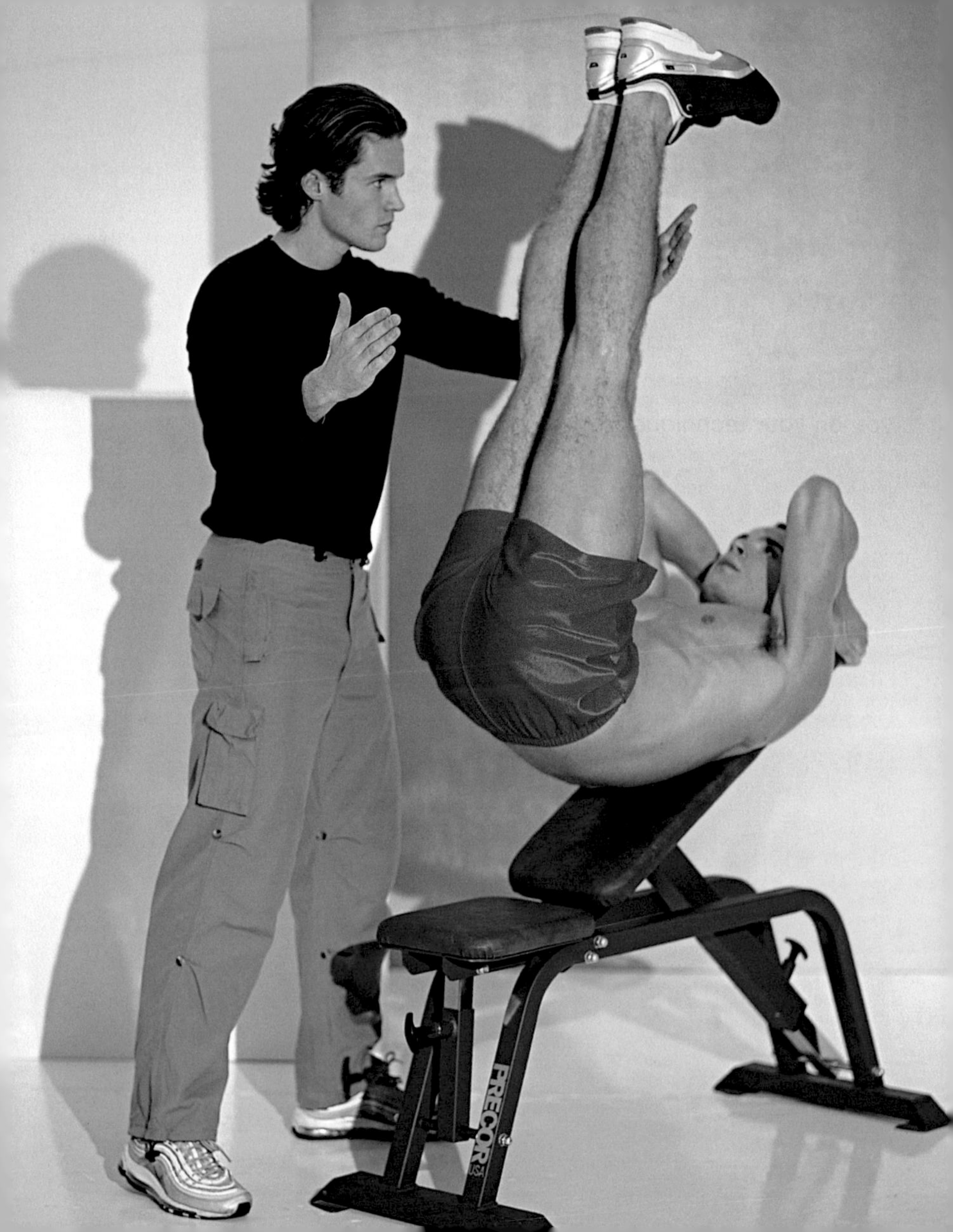
PRECOR
USA

here are exactly that. Secondly, you need a healthy, well-rounded diet: you'll find pointers on what to eat, what not to eat, and – just as importantly – when to eat throughout the book. Lastly, you need a cardio training routine that burns calories fast. I've given you guidelines for that too.

Alongside all this, I'll be passing on answers to those questions my clients ask me most about six-packs, advising you on your technique, and giving you suggestions for working out beyond the programme.

So grab your sports bag and head for the gym. The workouts take only about 20 minutes each. Do one every other day (keeping them in the same running order as they appear in the book), clean up your diet, and you should start to see results in a matter of weeks. Prepare for the testing prods of the envious!

workout one

First things first. To give your abs a good base of strength and tone, we'll focus on the central part of your stomach to start with.

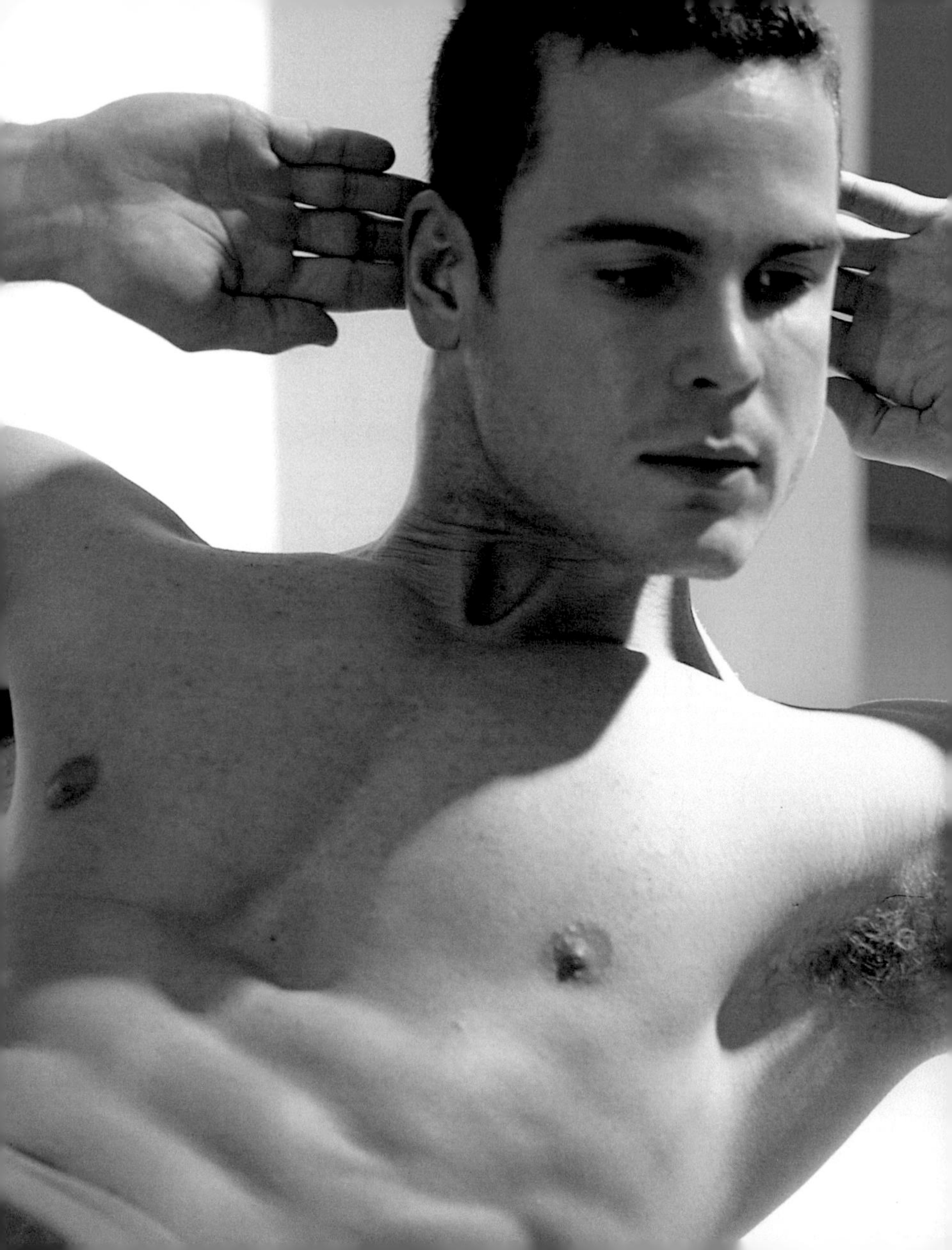

cardio

warm-up

Before you start the exercises in workout one, you need to warm up for 5–10 minutes on a piece of CV kit. The rower or cross-trainer is best as they work your upper body as well as your legs. You're not looking to kill yourself here, but you should start to raise a sweat.

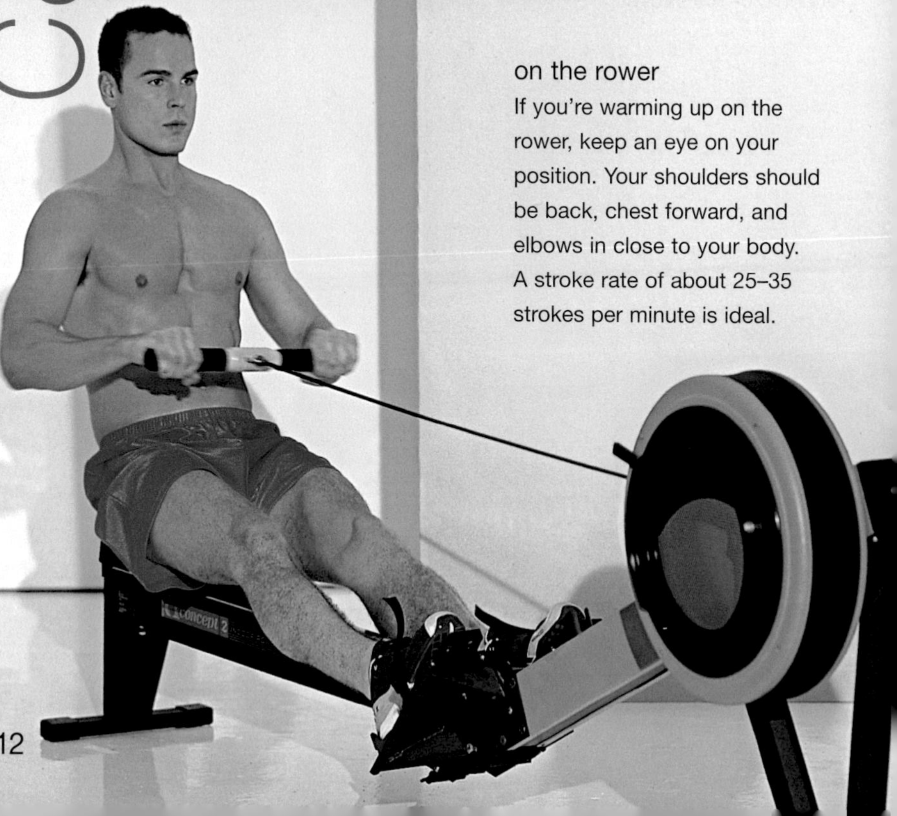

on the rower

If you're warming up on the rower, keep an eye on your position. Your shoulders should be back, chest forward, and elbows in close to your body. A stroke rate of about 25–35 strokes per minute is ideal.

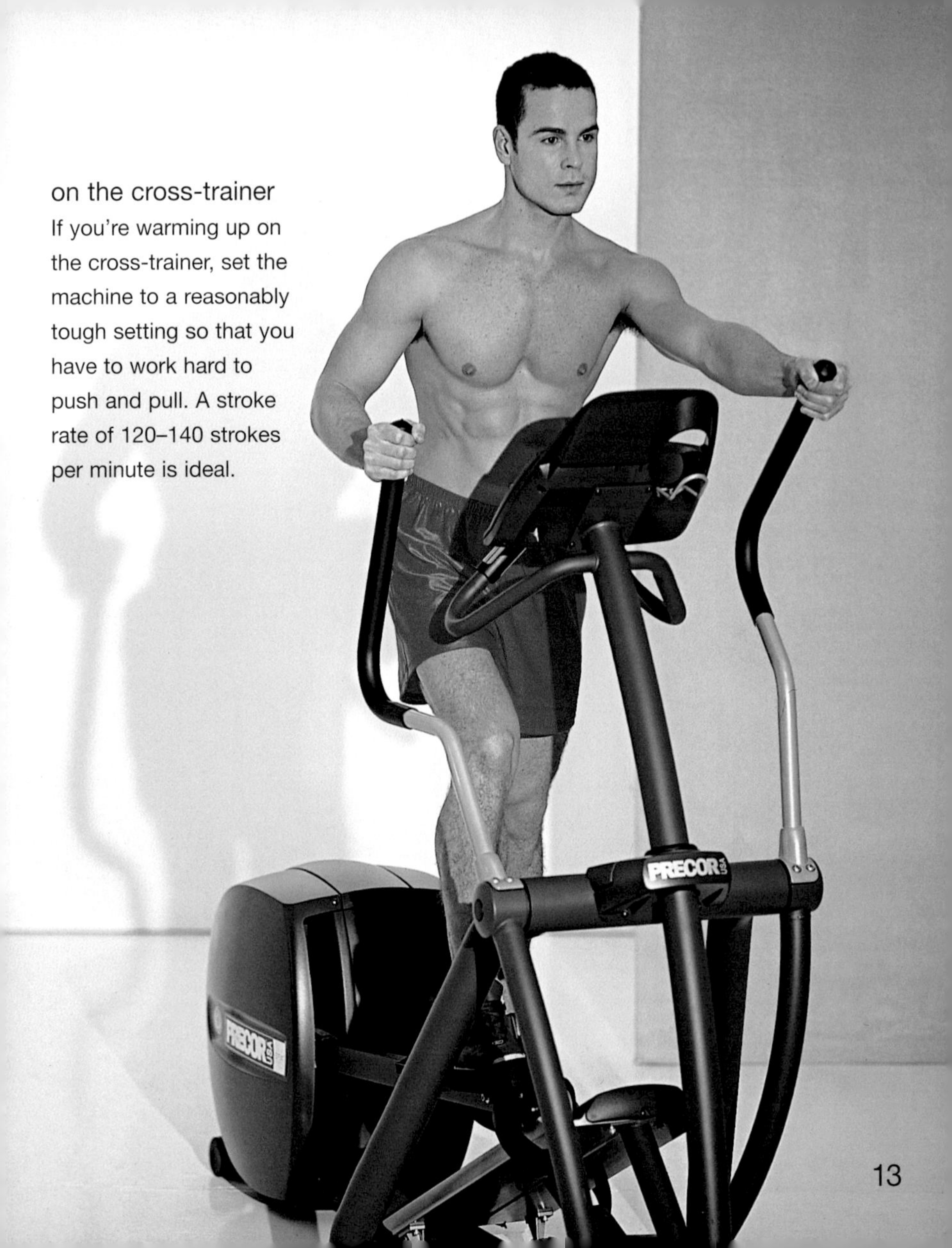

on the cross-trainer

If you're warming up on the cross-trainer, set the machine to a reasonably tough setting so that you have to work hard to push and pull. A stroke rate of 120–140 strokes per minute is ideal.

basic

sit-up

First up is the sit-up, but it's not the familiar exercise of old. Here, you curl your upper body no further forward than about 25° – the point at which your abs stop contracting and your hip muscles take over. Keep the movement slow and controlled so you can focus on getting your technique right. Each rep should take about 3–4 seconds.

level ①* do 20 reps

level ②* do 40 reps

1 Lie with your back in a comfortable 'neutral' position (don't flatten it into the floor or exaggerate its arch). Bend your knees and place your hands by your ears.

* check your level on page 92

2 Keeping your lower back on the floor and your abs tense, curl your shoulders forwards. Keep a space the size of an apple under your chin so your head stays in line with your spine. Slowly return to the start. After your last rep, move straight on to the next exercise.

do it right

breathing check

Breathing correctly is an important part of effective training. Get into the habit of breathing in just before you move and breathing out as you move. With most of the exercises, one full in-and-out breath per rep is right.

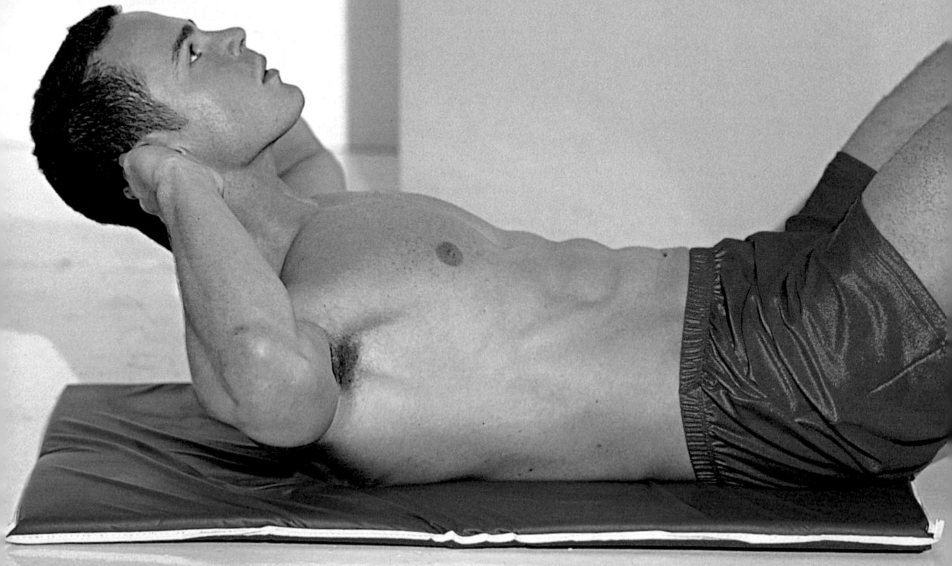

reverse curl

A great exercise to stimulate your abs from the lower end. Focus on using them to pull your pelvis and legs towards you, rather than throwing your legs over your head. Take about 3–4 seconds per rep.

level ① do 20 reps

level ② do 30 reps

1 Lie on your back with your hands behind your head and your legs straight up in the air. Keep your shoulders and head on the floor throughout.

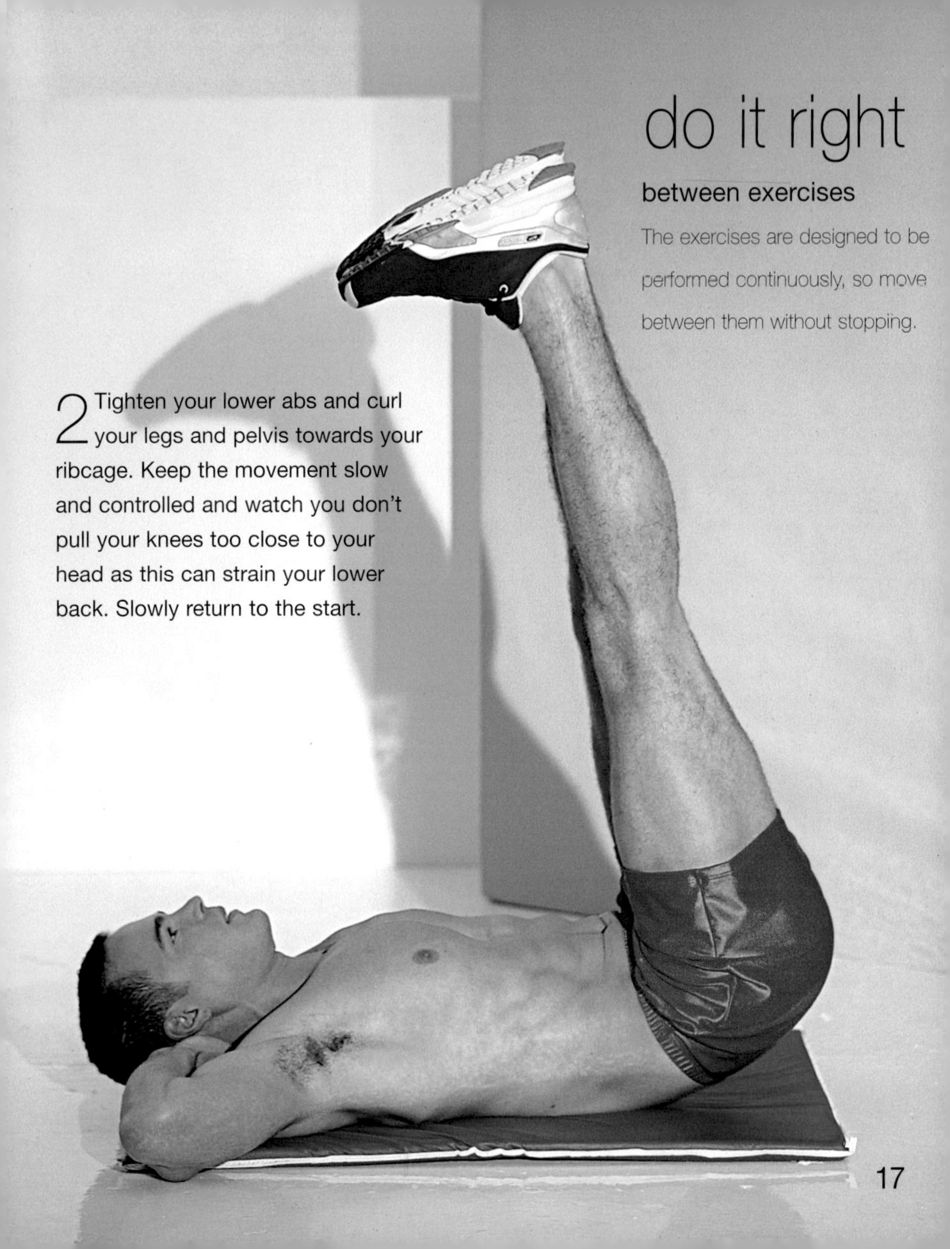

do it right

between exercises

The exercises are designed to be performed continuously, so move between them without stopping.

2 Tighten your lower abs and curl your legs and pelvis towards your ribcage. Keep the movement slow and controlled and watch you don't pull your knees too close to your head as this can strain your lower back. Slowly return to the start.

oblique crunch

This crunch targets your obliques – the muscles at the sides of your waist.

level ① do 20 reps per side

level ② do 30 reps per side

1 Lie on your back with your knees bent, your feet flat on the floor, and your hands by your ears.

2 Raise one shoulder and one elbow up towards your opposite knee. Slowly return to the start position. For the next rep, raise your other shoulder and elbow. Then work alternate sides.

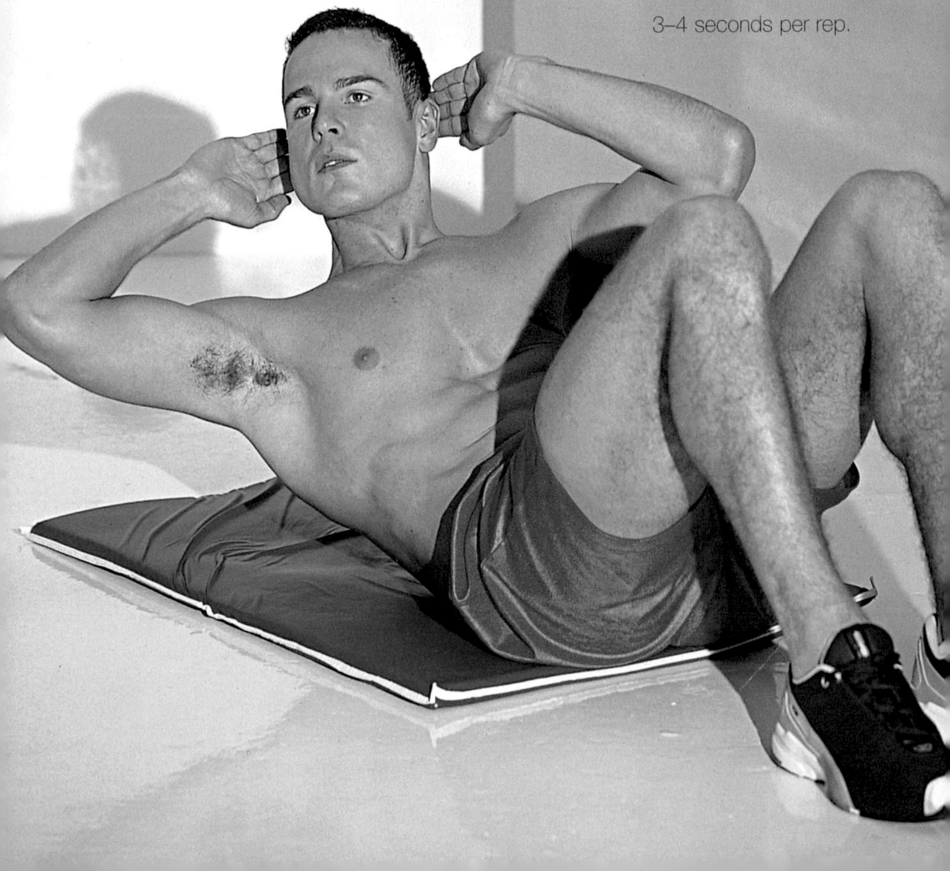

do it right

rep speed

The exact time each rep should take you varies from exercise to exercise, but as a rough rule of thumb allow 3–4 seconds per rep.

full crunch

One of the most advanced exercises for your abs. This combines the movements of the basic sit-up with the movements of the reverse curl. It works your entire stomach area.

level ① do 20 reps

level ② do 40 reps

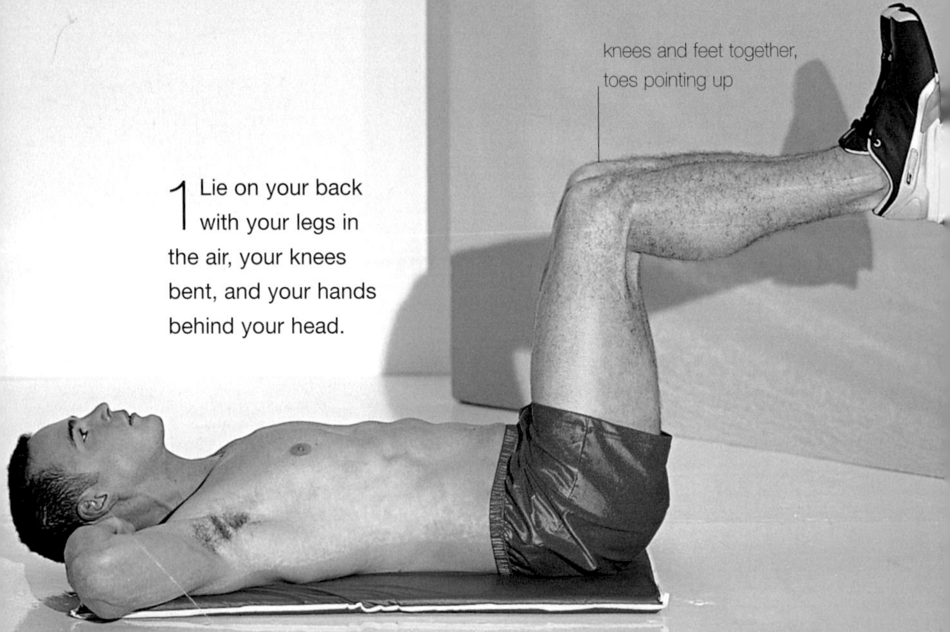

knees and feet together, toes pointing up

1 Lie on your back with your legs in the air, your knees bent, and your hands behind your head.

2 Curl your legs and pelvis towards your ribcage. At the same time, curl your shoulders forwards. Watch you don't tense the muscles of your neck. Slowly return to the start position.

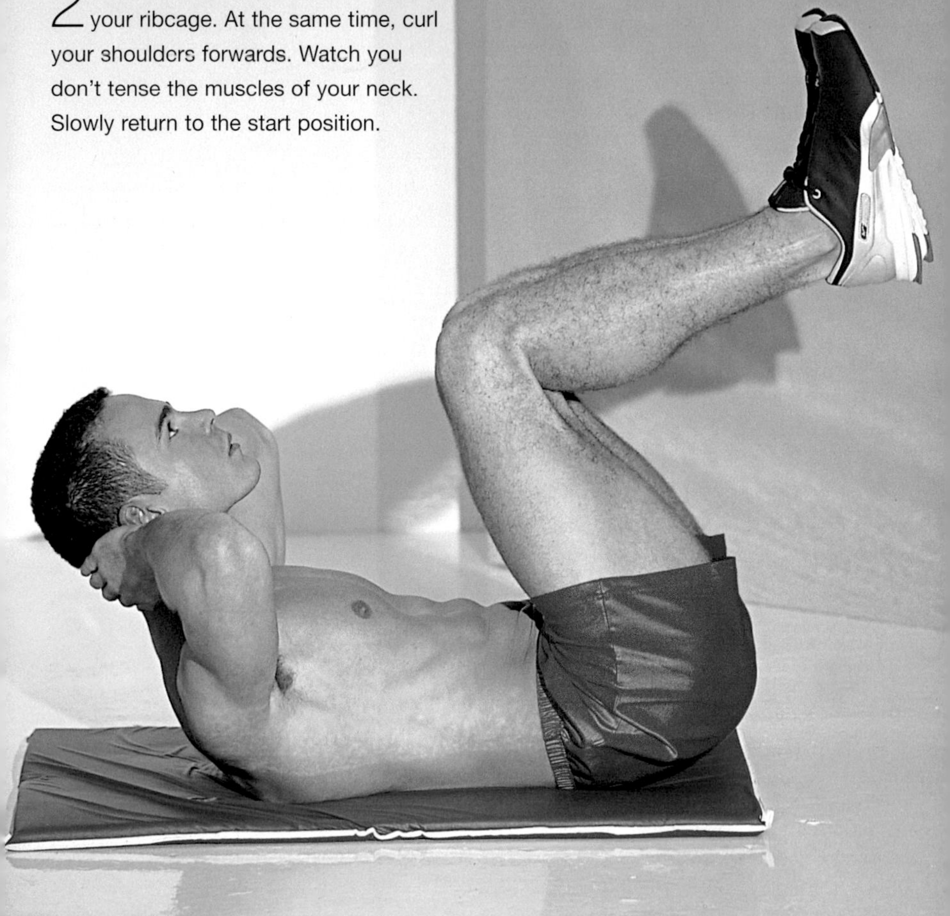

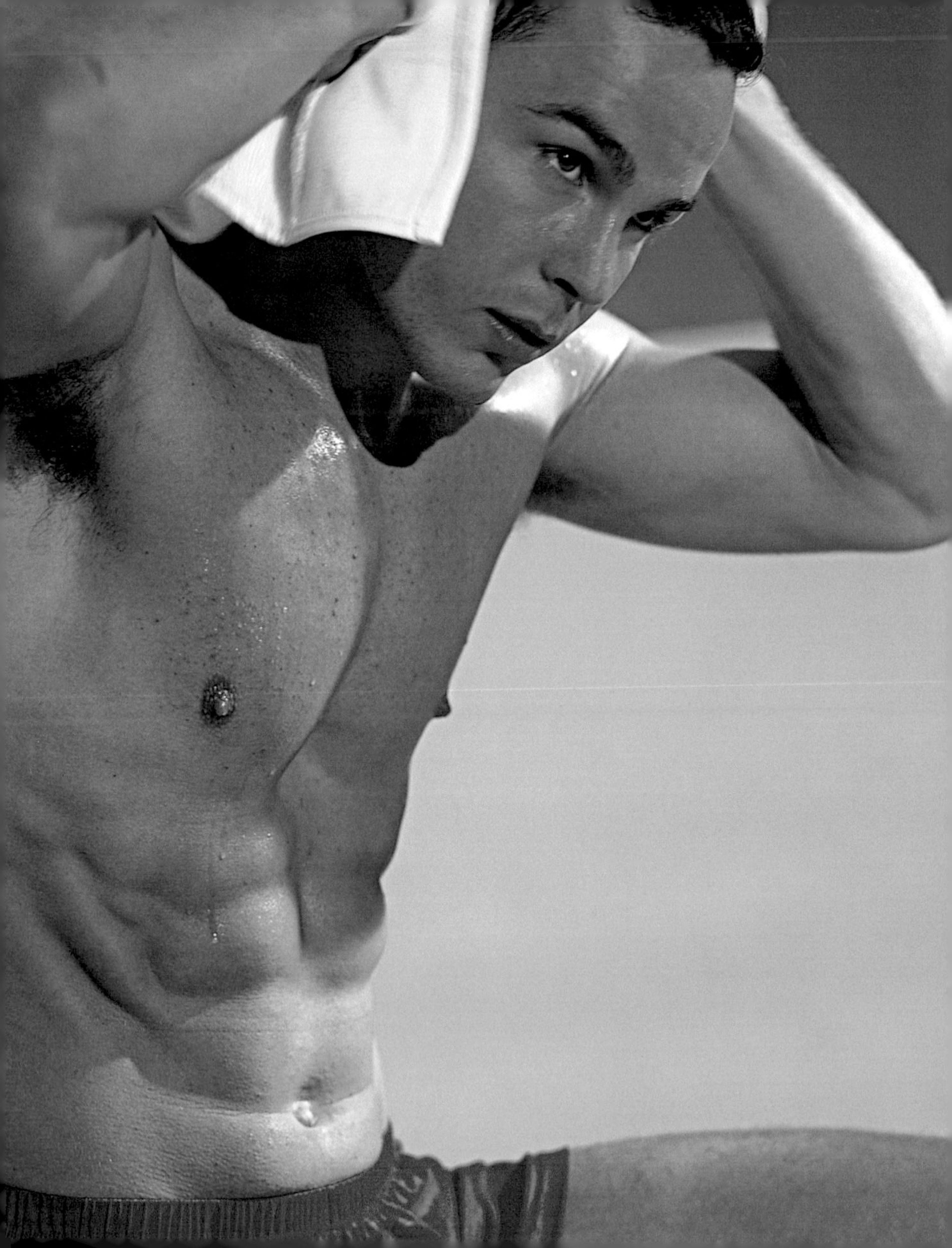

You'll have got the hang of my approach now – to blitz the muscles of your abdomen from every conceivable angle. It's a technique that gives good returns fast, believe me.

reverse curl crunch

A slightly different combination of the basic sit-up and the reverse curl, and one of the most effective ways to work your stomach. The movements may be fairly small, but the effects are great.

level ① do 20 reps

level ② do 30 reps

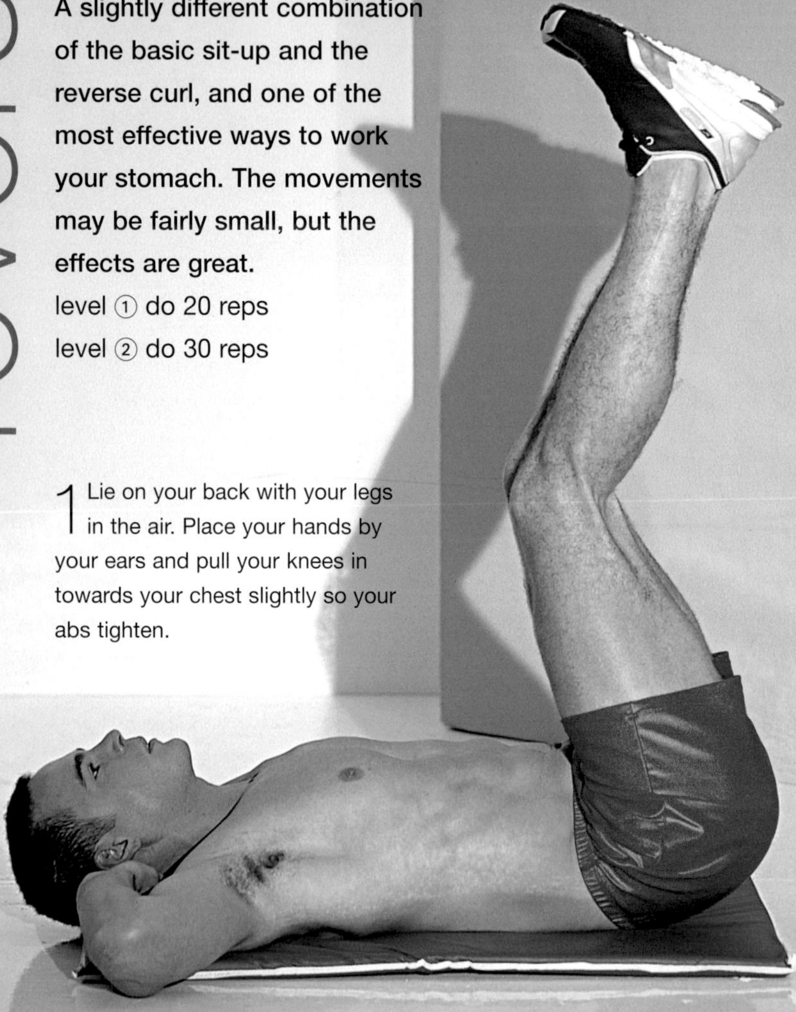

1 Lie on your back with your legs in the air. Place your hands by your ears and pull your knees in towards your chest slightly so your abs tighten.

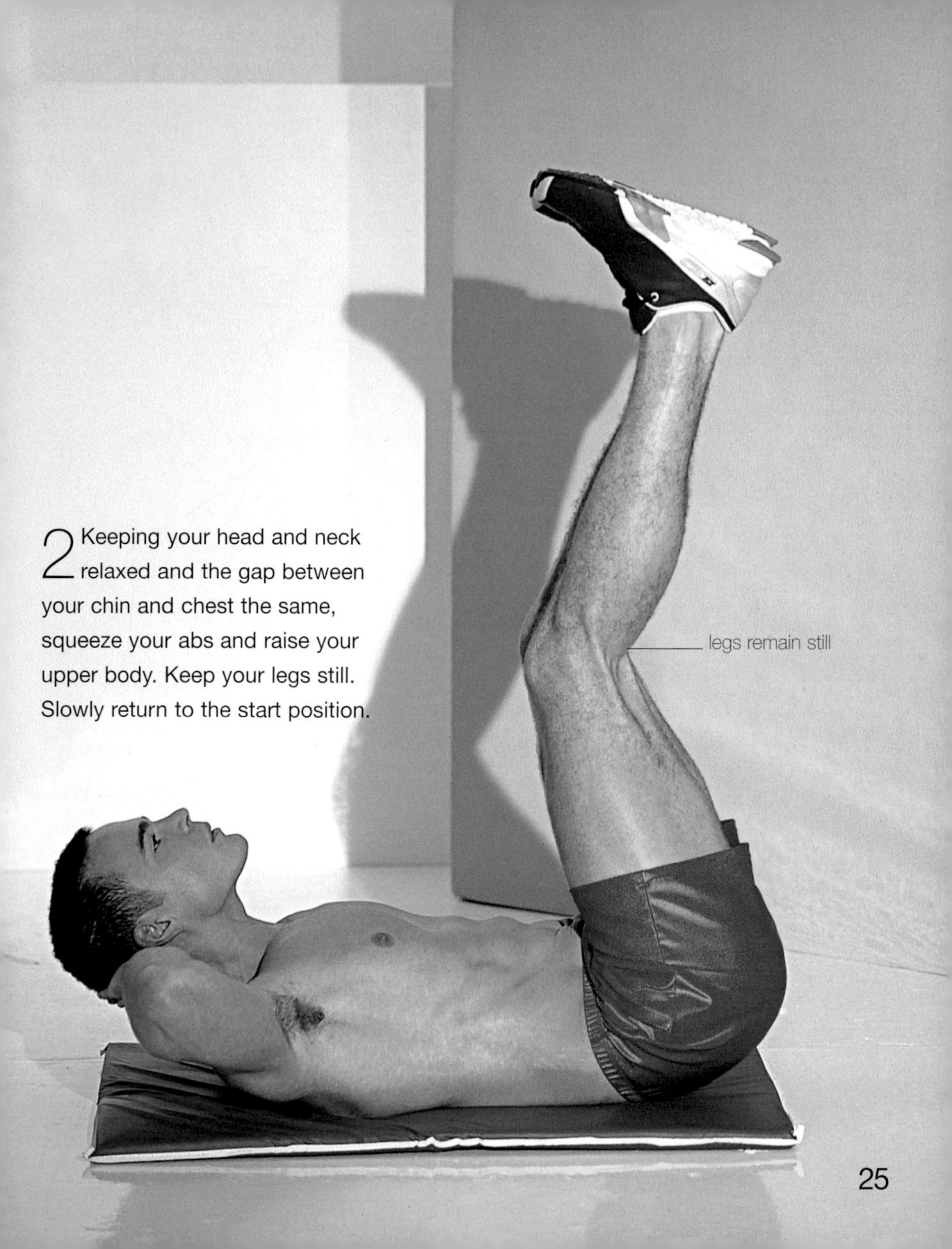

2 Keeping your head and neck relaxed and the gap between your chin and chest the same, squeeze your abs and raise your upper body. Keep your legs still. Slowly return to the start position.

legs remain still

oblique

knee pull

A good exercise for your obliques (though the whole of your abdominal area gets a massive workout too). Focus on them as the main working muscles.

level ① do 15 reps per side

level ② do 20 reps per side

1 Lie with your lower back in a comfortable neutral position. Keep one leg on the floor and raise your other leg so your thigh is at right angles to it. Place your hands by your ears, elbows bent out wide, shoulders down.

2 Squeezing your abs and pivoting on one elbow, bring your other elbow and shoulder towards your knee. At the same time, move your knee towards your elbow. Keep your elbow out wide and your hips on the floor. Slowly return to the start. Do all the knee pulls on one side, then switch to your other side.

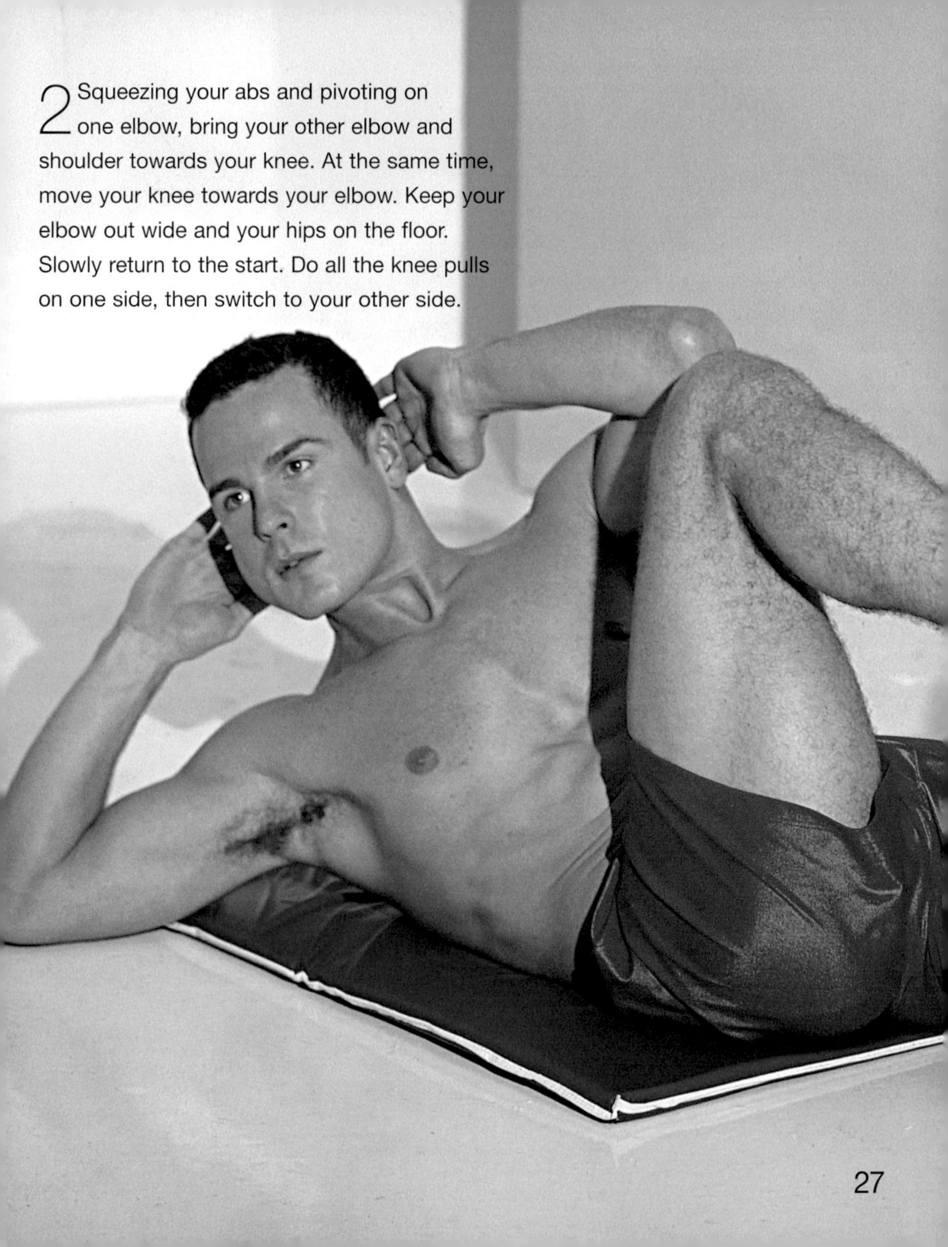

medicine ball sit-up

This sit-up with a medicine ball is tough because it gives greater loading on your stomach. Once you get the hang of it, try holding the ball with your hands extended over your head. That way, it's tougher still. **See page 90 for the exact position.**

level ① do 20 reps

level ② do 40 reps

1 Lie on your back with knees bent and feet flat on the floor. Hold a medicine ball to your chest with both hands.

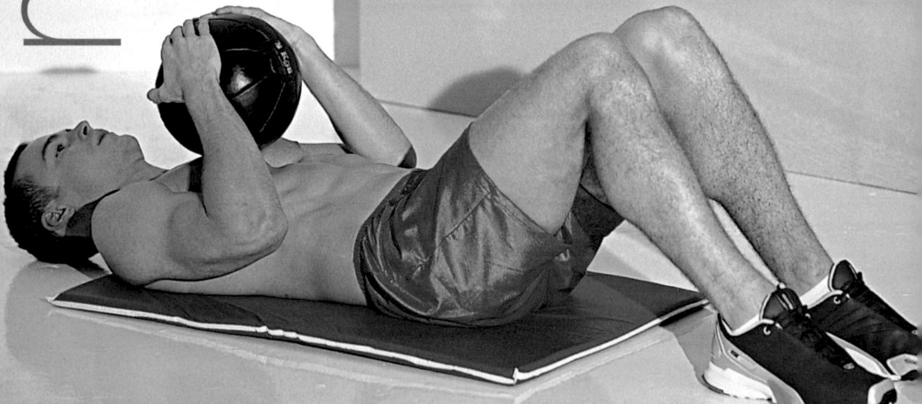

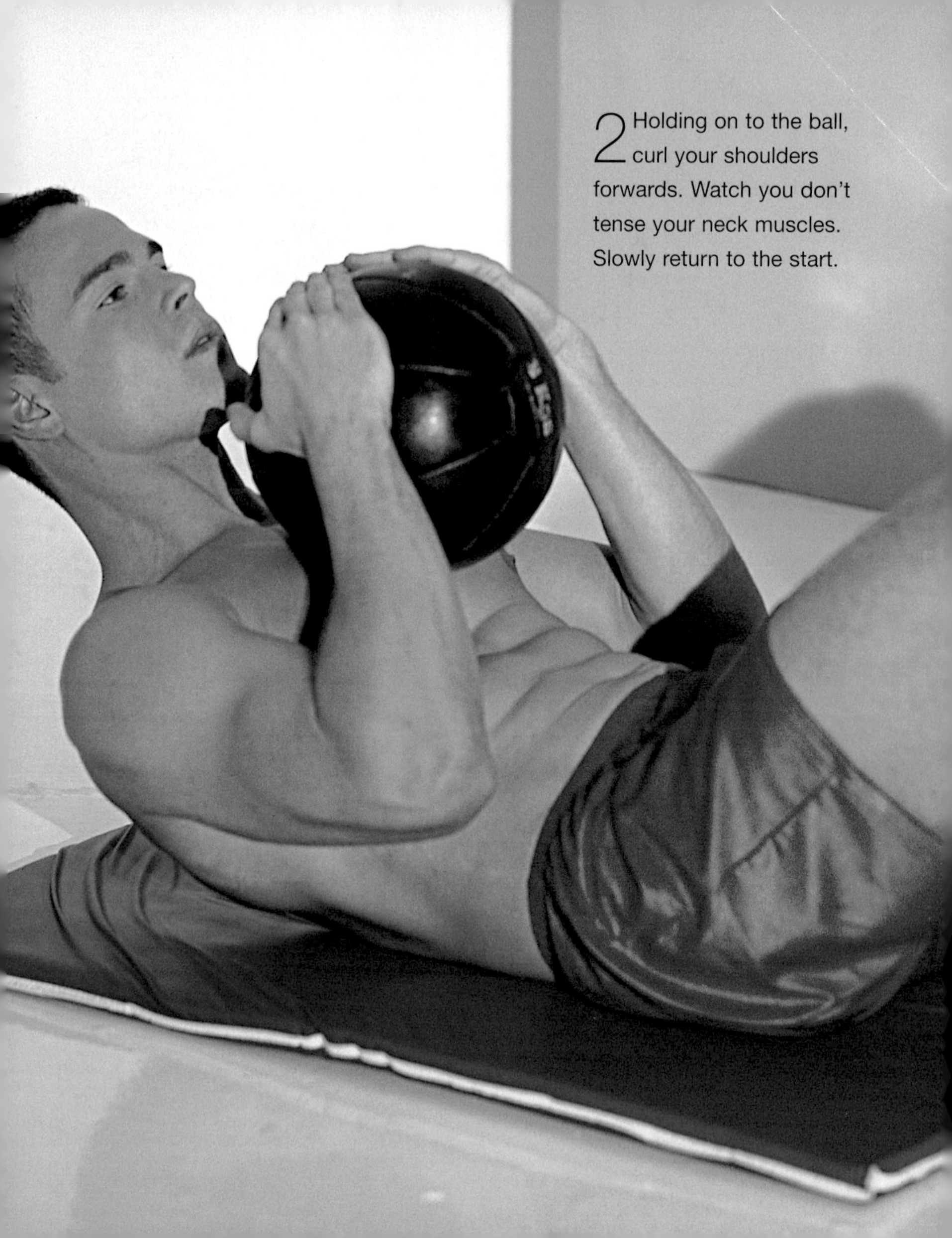

2 Holding on to the ball, curl your shoulders forwards. Watch you don't tense your neck muscles. Slowly return to the start.

essential stretches

You may feel your muscles don't need stretching right now, but 5 minutes' work will ward off nagging back problems later. Do these stretch moves in order.

1 hip flexor

Kneel on both knees, then step forwards with one foot. Keep your other knee on the floor. Rest your hands on the extended knee. Slide your back leg out behind you. Feel the stretch in the front of your hip. Hold for 10–12 seconds. Repeat with your other leg.

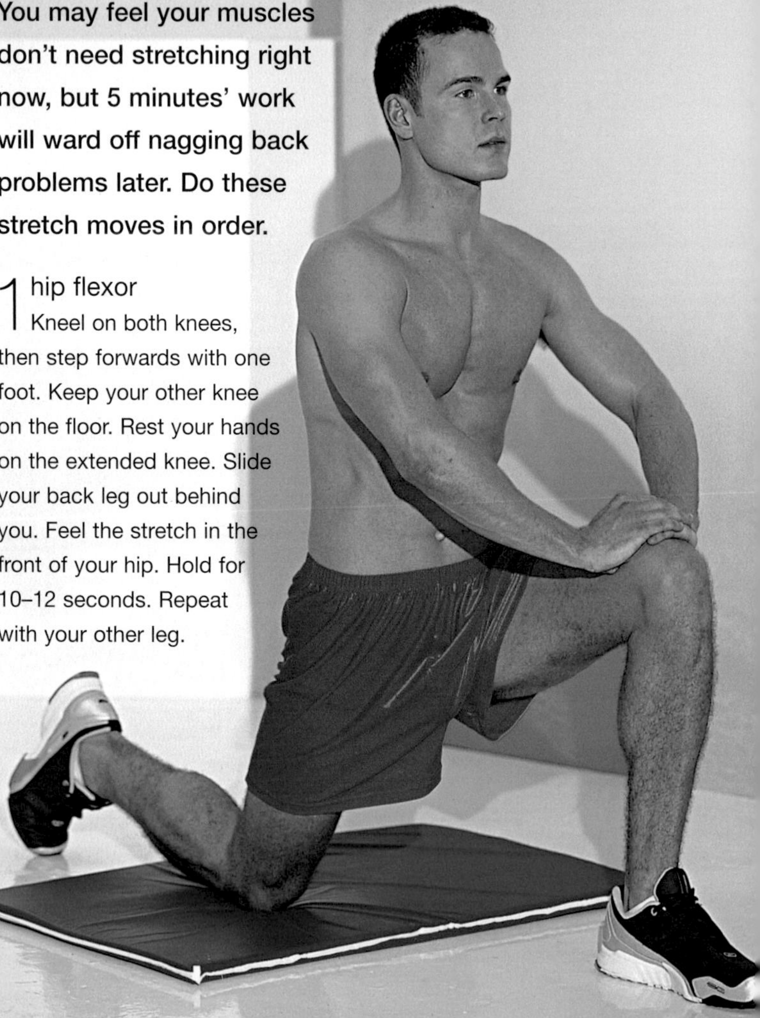

2 cobra stretch

Lie on your front with your elbows tucked in close to your body. Keeping your hips on the floor, push your torso up until you're supporting your upper body on your elbows and forearms. Keep your neck relaxed. Hold for 15 seconds, then slowly return to the start position.

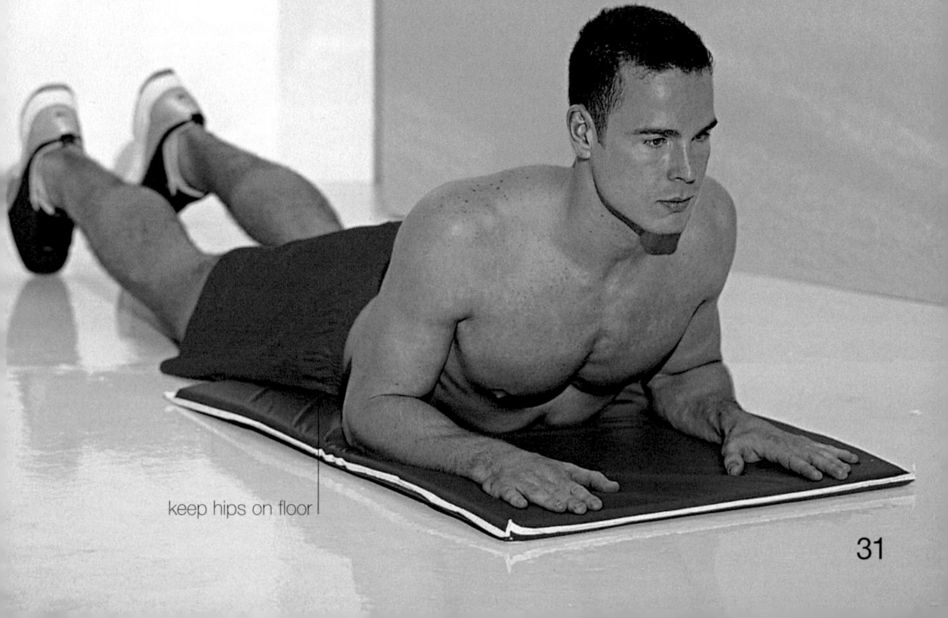

keep hips on floor

3 cat stretch

Position yourself on your hands and knees, with your back straight. Push your spine upwards to create a curve in the middle of your back. Hold for 5 seconds, then slowly return to the start position.

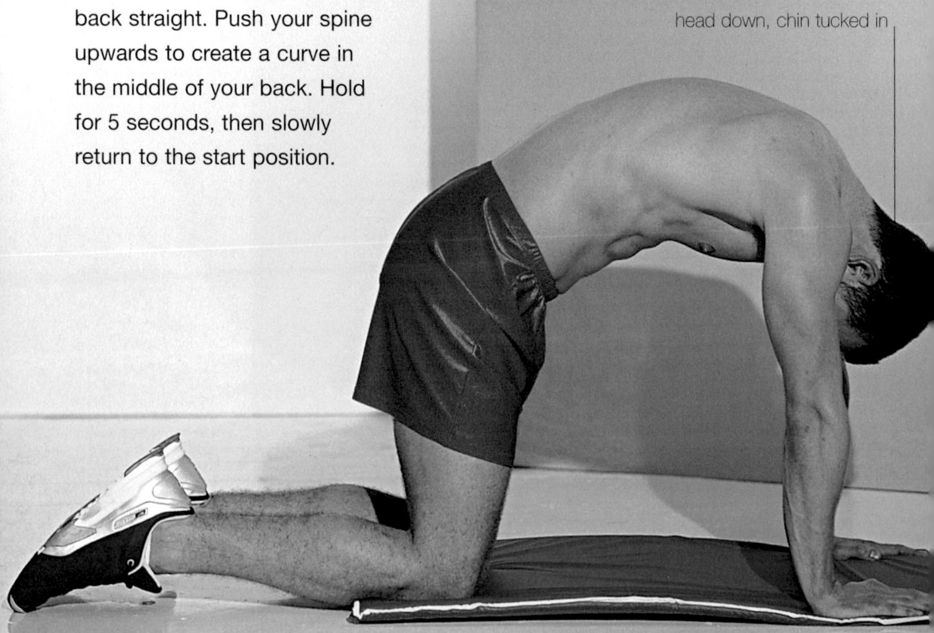

head down, chin tucked in

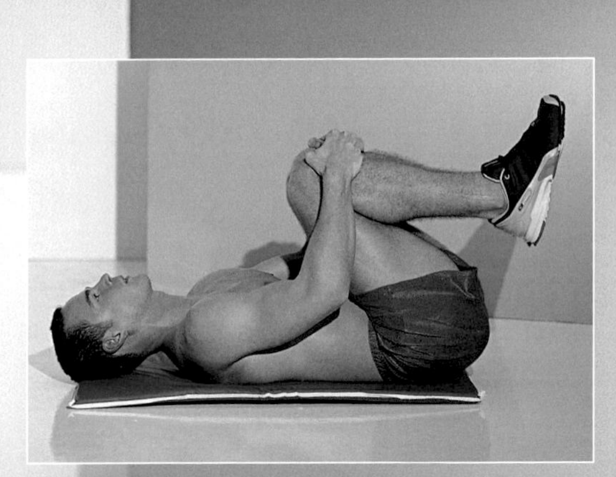

5 lower back stretch

Still lying down, hold the tops of your shins with both hands. Gently pull your knees in close to your body until you can feel the stretch in your lower back. Hold for 10 seconds, then slowly return to the start.

4 spine rotation

Lie down and stretch your arms out at shoulder level. Bend both legs to 90°, then drop your knees to the side so one knee is touching the floor. Keep your shoulder blades flat on the floor, but don't force the stretch. Hold for 15 seconds, then slowly return to the start position. Repeat on your other side.

Q&A

ab blasters

I do a hundred sit-ups a day, so how come I don't I have a flat stomach?

This is a question I'm always being asked and I usually give the same answer. Check your technique first of all: the quality of the exercise is as important as the number of reps you're doing. Secondly, make sure you're 'overloading' your stomach muscles (increasing the demands you're making on them) by targeting them from several different angles. You won't be able to do this with sit-ups alone, but the combination of exercises I've put together in this book should work like a dream. And remember that your abs – like any other muscle – can be overtrained. Always allow at least a day between ab workouts.

I've got a layer of fat on my abs that I just can't shift. What can I do to get rid of it?

I think you could do with giving your diet the once-over. Exercise on its own is no guarantee you'll end up with a perfect six-pack. What's more, it's nigh on impossible to lose fat from just one area of your body. So make sure you follow the nutrition tips I've given you in the book. Get into the habit of watching what you eat and when you eat it. And start taking some regular cardio exercise (*see opposite*).

Do I need to do exercises for my lower back while I'm working on my abs?

Good point. Your midsection is a bit like a cylinder, I always think, with your abs at the front, your *erector spinae* at the back, and your obliques at the sides. Each of these areas is as important as the rest, and for balance in your midsection – indeed throughout your entire body – you need to work them equally. There's no need to worry about this while you're doing the workouts in this book – I've taken care of it in my choice of exercises.

Should I incorporate cardio work into my exercise routine?

Yes, you should. It's essential, in fact. Successful ab training is a combination of three things: a good ab workout (you have three of them in this book), a healthy diet, and regular cardio work. Follow this formula to a T and you should have the low body fat you need to show off a well-chiselled six-pack. In terms of cardio work, do a little extra rowing or cross-training, or hit the treadmill and either run or walk on an incline.

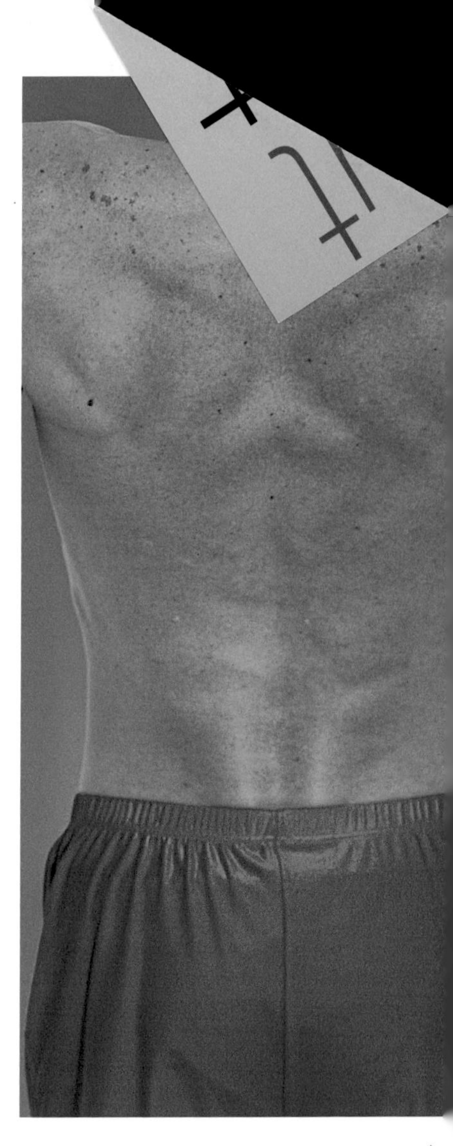

workout two

Time to shift the focus of attention to your obliques now. As all trace of 'love handles' disappears, a more 'corseted', defined you should emerge.

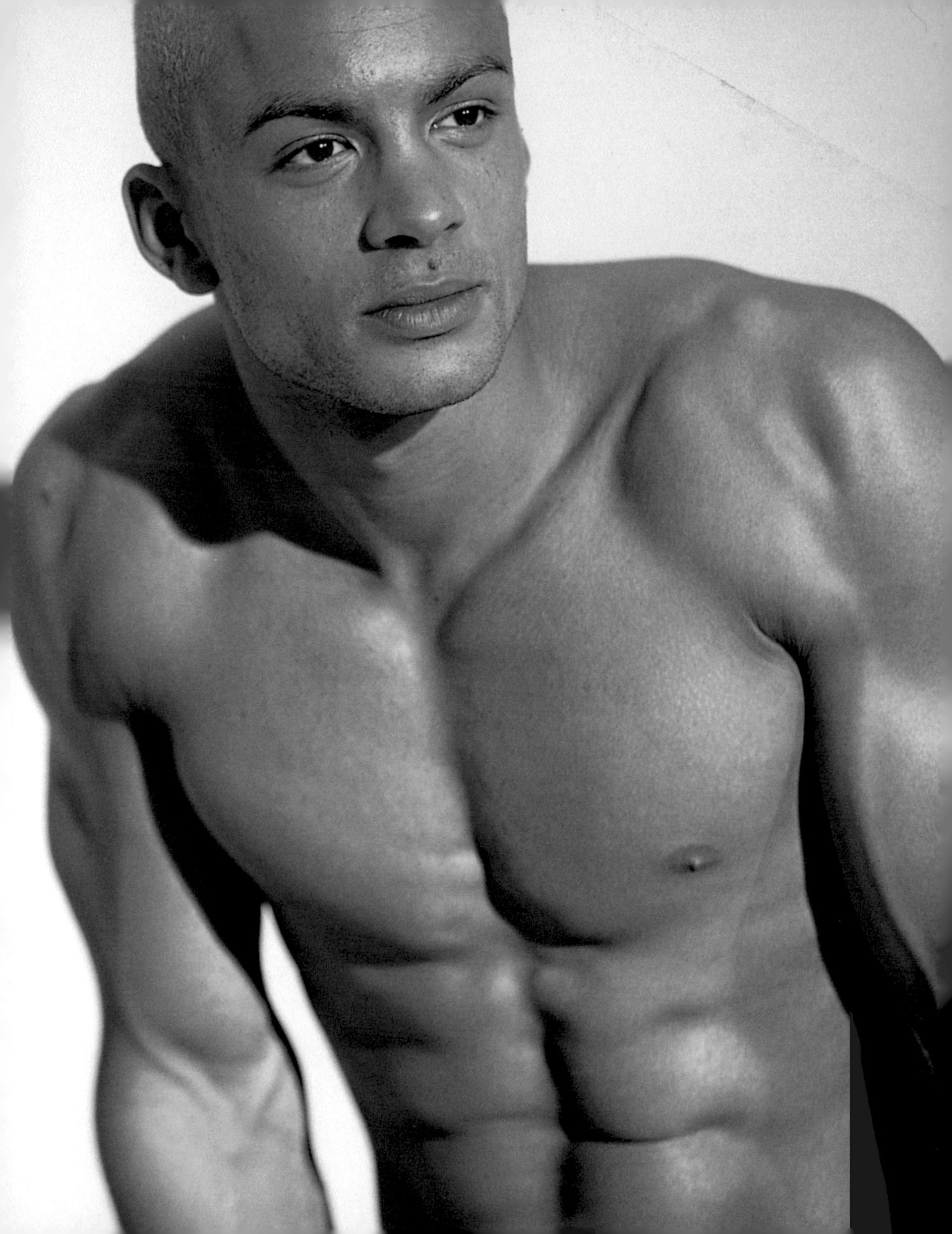

cardio warm-up

If you decide to warm up on the rower, take care to generate most of the stroke power from your legs. And keep a relaxed grip on the handle so your forearms don't tire too quickly. Again, a stroke rate of 25–35 strokes per minute is ideal.

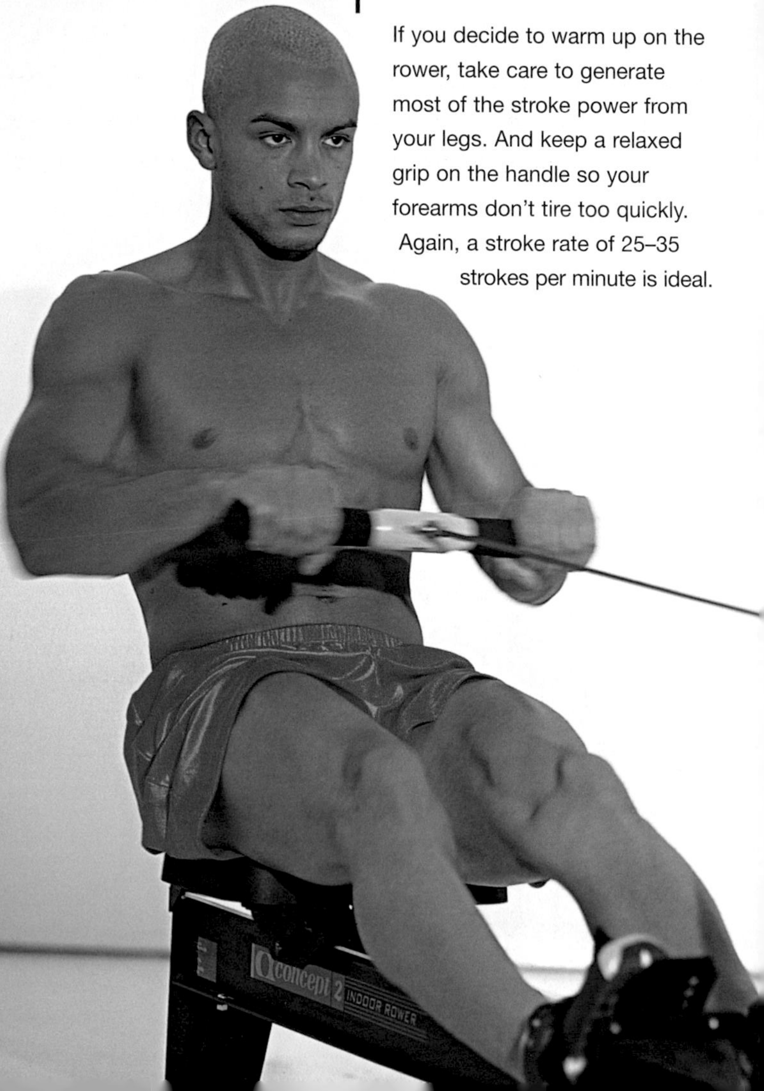

Before you get down to the exercises in workout two, you need to warm up on a piece of CV kit for 5–10 minutes, just as you did before workout one. Again, the choice is yours – the rower or cross-trainer. Remember, you're not looking to kill yourself. But you should start to raise a sweat.

extended leg crunch

With this exercise, make sure you keep your extended leg completely still so you intensify the loading on your abdomen and obliques.

level ① do 15 reps per leg

level ② do 20 reps per leg

1 Lie on your back with one foot flat on the floor and the other leg extended in front of you just below the height of your adjacent knee. Place your hands by your ears and spread your elbows out wide.

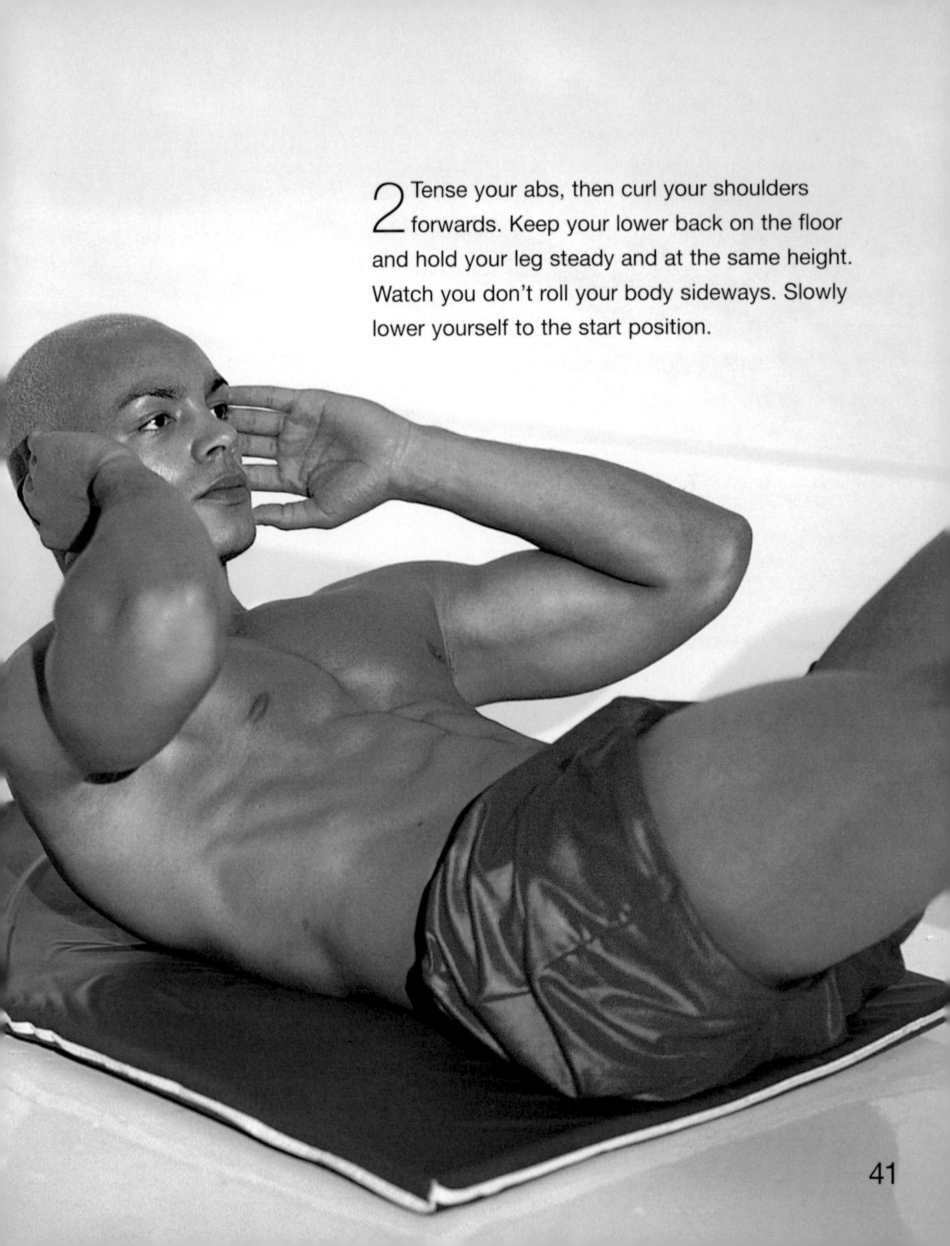

2 Tense your abs, then curl your shoulders forwards. Keep your lower back on the floor and hold your leg steady and at the same height. Watch you don't roll your body sideways. Slowly lower yourself to the start position.

straight leg crunch

The crucial thing with this exercise is the position of your body: make sure you keep your pelvis tilted towards you and your lower back pressed in to the floor. That way, you won't be able to bow your back and injure it. Perform the crunch very slowly.

level ① do 20 reps

level ② do 30 reps

1 Lie on your back with your legs extended in front of you, feet together. Press your lower back into the floor so your pelvis tilts towards you. Place your hands by your ears.

2 Tense your abs and curl your upper body forwards, one vertebra at a time. Make sure your lower back stays in contact with the floor and keep your neck relaxed. Slowly return to the start position.

bridge

This is a static hold that has its roots in yoga. Don't be fooled by how easy it looks – it will test your stomach muscles to the limit and force you to use a massive range of muscle groups.

level ① hold for 30 secs

level ② hold for 60 secs

1 Position yourself with your toes on the floor and your elbows directly below your shoulders.

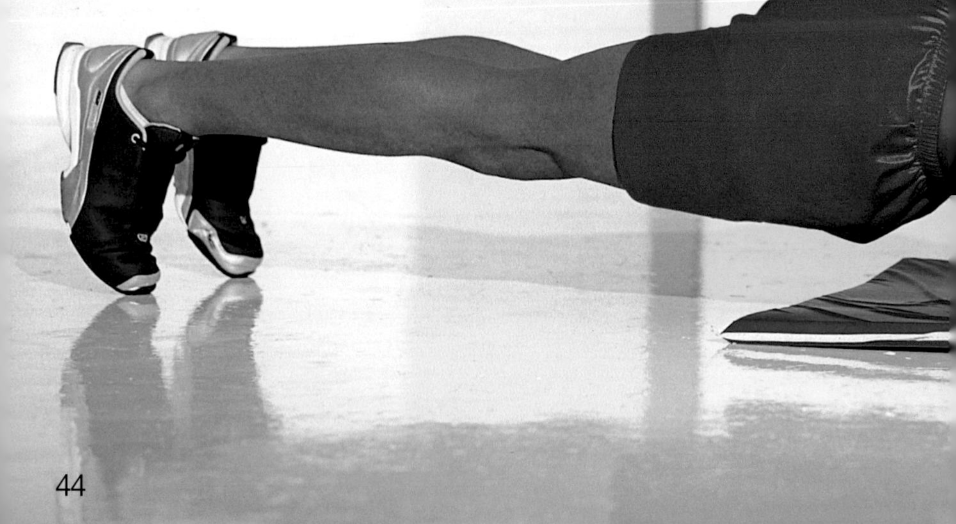

2 Keeping a straight line from your shoulders to your ankles, raise yourself up so your elbows, forearms, and toes support your body. Use your abs to maintain the position. Slowly return to the start.

keep your body straight

eat lean

lose the love handles

Whether you're sculpting a six-pack *and* trying to lose a few pounds or simply looking after the one you already have, it pays to eat lean. After all, your stomach's usually the first place to let you know you've put on a bit of weight.

- Avoid starchy foods such as wheat products and potatoes.
- Eat grilled, roasted, or steamed food and leave the fried stuff well alone.
- Drink at least 2 litres (3½ pints) of water every day. It helps flush impurities through your system.
- And cut out alcohol or reduce your intake to 8 units a week at the very most.

full crunch

A favourite fallback exercise of mine that's guaranteed to work your abs hard. Keep your mind focused firmly on them as you crunch into a ball.

level ① do 20 reps

level ② do 40 reps

1 Lie on your back with your legs in the air and your knees bent. Place your hands on either side of your head by your ears.

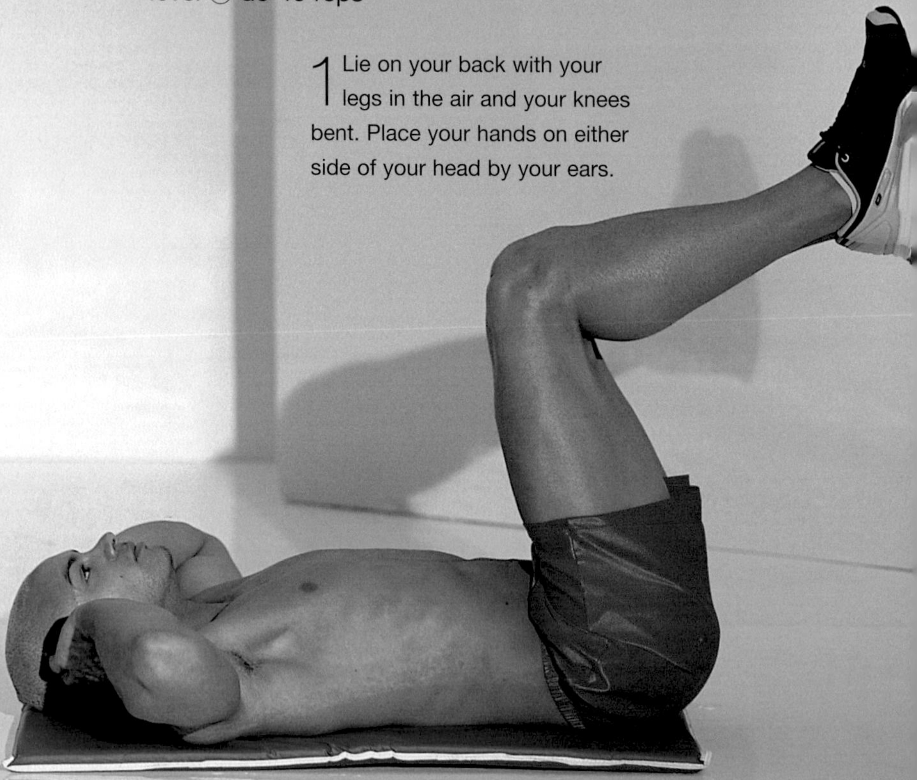

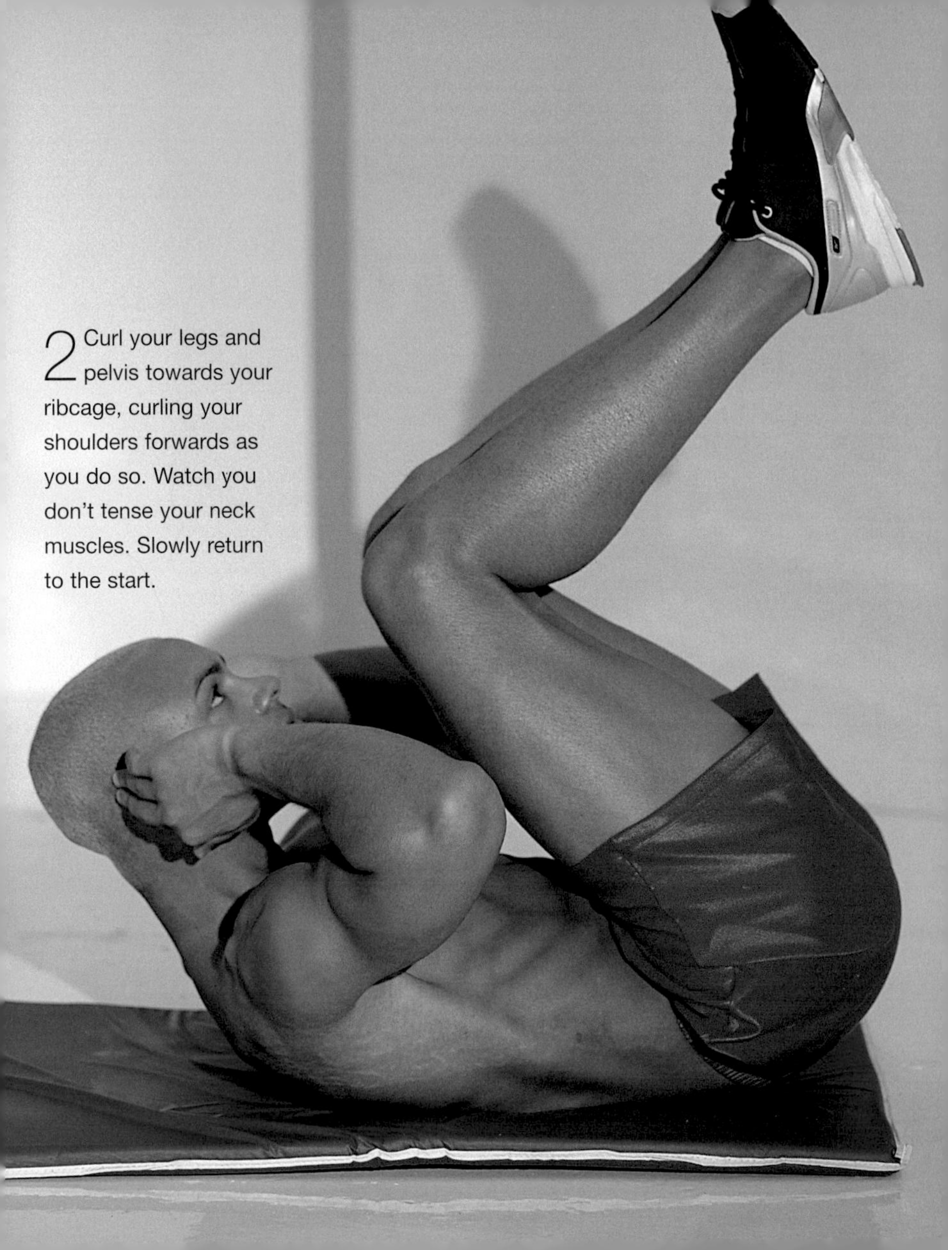

2 Curl your legs and pelvis towards your ribcage, curling your shoulders forwards as you do so. Watch you don't tense your neck muscles. Slowly return to the start.

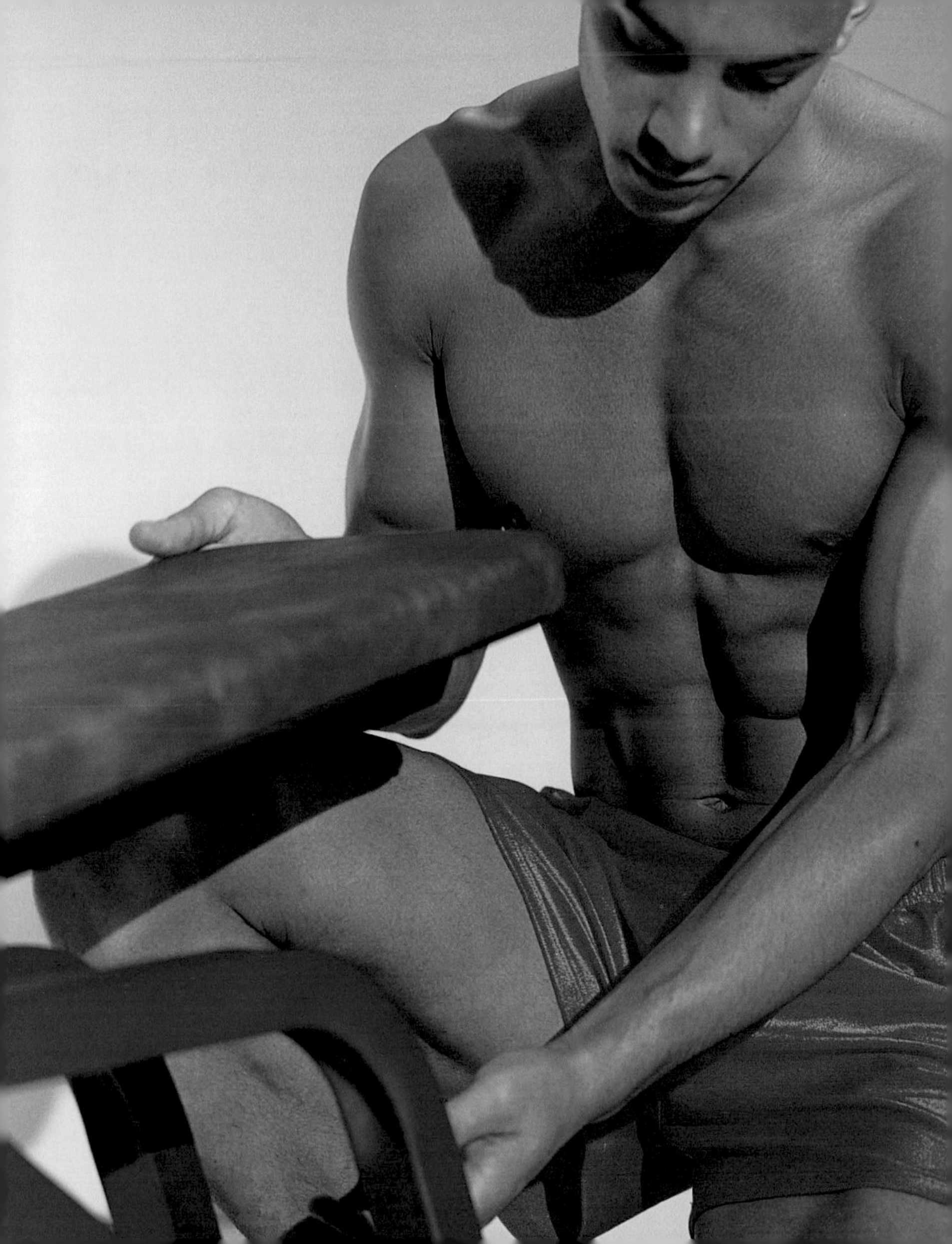

It's all too easy to go through the motions during a workout and end up way off target. Focus on the area you're working. Concentrate on getting the exercises spot on. The results of good technique far outstrip those you get with a sloppy approach.

bench

reverse curl

A real show stopper this one. But performed well, it works your abs hard. Just hang on tight.

level ① do 15 reps

level ② do 30 reps

1 Lie on the bench with the top end raised to about 45°. Hold the top of the bench to keep your body steady. Start with your legs slightly bent and your feet in the air.

2 Tighten your lower abs and, lifting your lower back off the bench, curl your legs and pelvis towards your ribcage. Hold for 1 second, then slowly return to the start position.

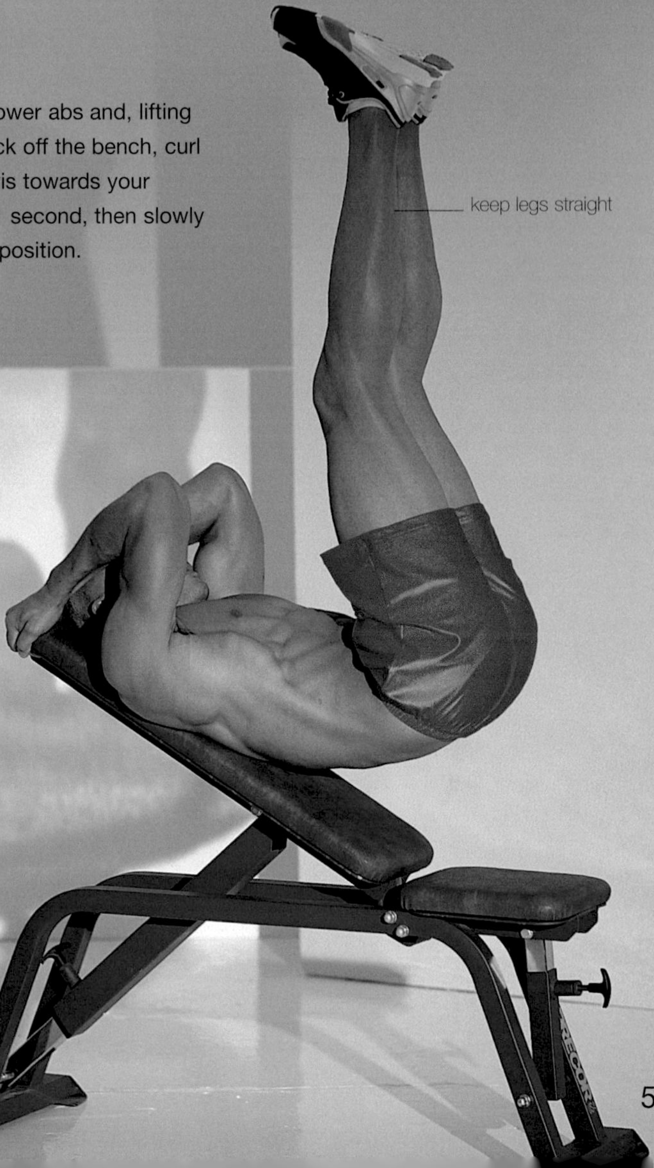

keep legs straight

oblique bridge

Static work is tough, as you've already found out with the basic bridge. This exercise tests your obliques from all angles.

level ① hold for 30 secs per side

level ② hold for 60 secs per side

1 Lie on your side with your elbow and forearm directly under your shoulder as support. Rest your other hand on your stomach. Place one foot on top of the other.

2 Raise yourself up, keeping a straight line from your head to your toes. Maintain the position by using your obliques (the muscles at the sides of your stomach). Slowly lower yourself to the start position.

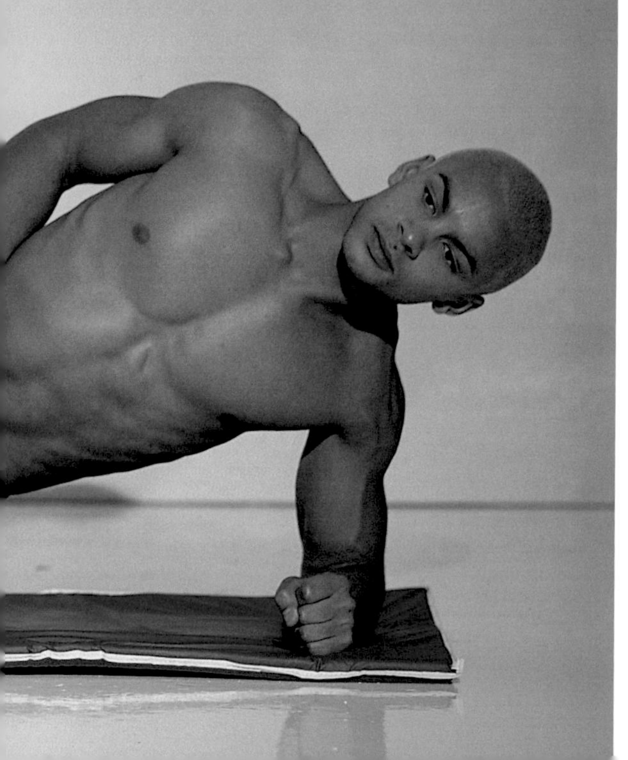

eat lean

six-pack friendly foods

Unless mother nature has been exceptionally kind to you, your dream of owning a set of chiselled abs without keeping an eye on what you eat is unlikely ever to amount to more than a dream. There's no getting away from the fact that diet plays a vital role in defining your mid-section. You're probably all too familiar with what you shouldn't eat (just in case you aren't, there's a run-down on page 83), so here's a list of six-pack friendly fare you can enjoy: chicken, turkey, firm white fish, tuna, wholemeal pasta, brown rice, dishes made from pulses (like kidney beans or lentils), and almost any fruit and veg.

single-knee crunch

After the last few exercises, your obliques might well need some assistance. Your abdominals come to the rescue here.

level ① do 20 reps per leg

level ② do 40 reps per leg

1 Lie on your back with your lower back pressed into the floor and your legs straight up in the air. Pull your head away from the floor slightly. Place your hands by your ears.

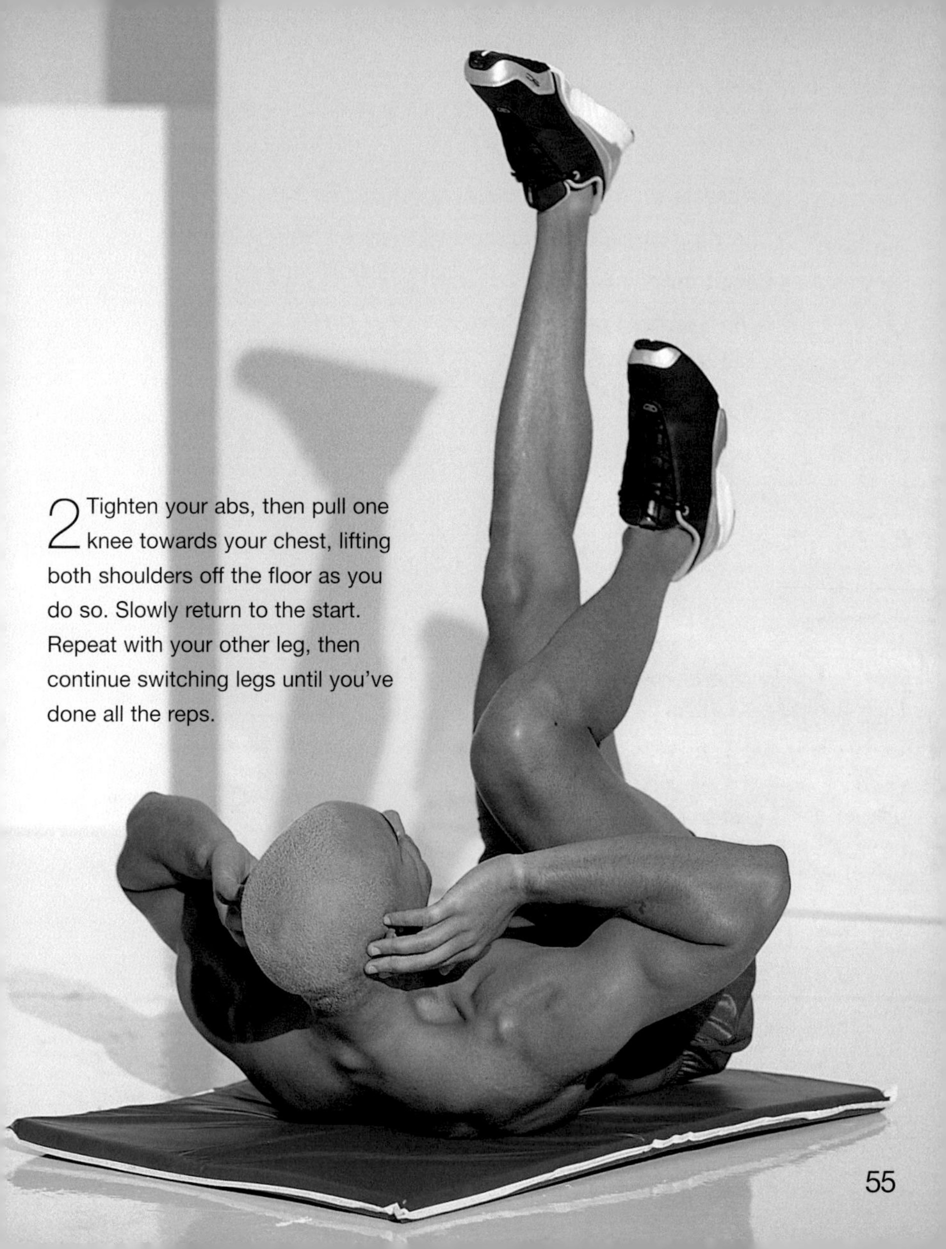

2 Tighten your abs, then pull one knee towards your chest, lifting both shoulders off the floor as you do so. Slowly return to the start. Repeat with your other leg, then continue switching legs until you've done all the reps.

oblique

bridge raise

This advance on the static oblique bridge makes the muscles in your stomach and at the sides of your waist dynamic and strong.

level ① do 15 reps per side

level ② do 30 reps per side

1 Lie on your side with your elbow and forearm directly under your shoulder as support. Rest the other hand on your stomach. Place one foot on the other, then raise yourself up, keeping a straight line from your head to your toes and maintaining the position with your obliques.

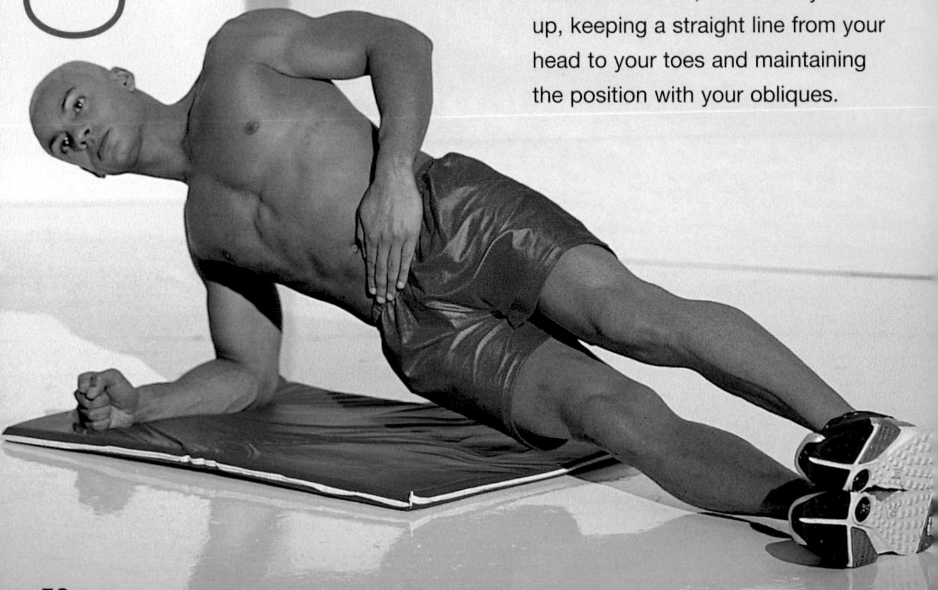

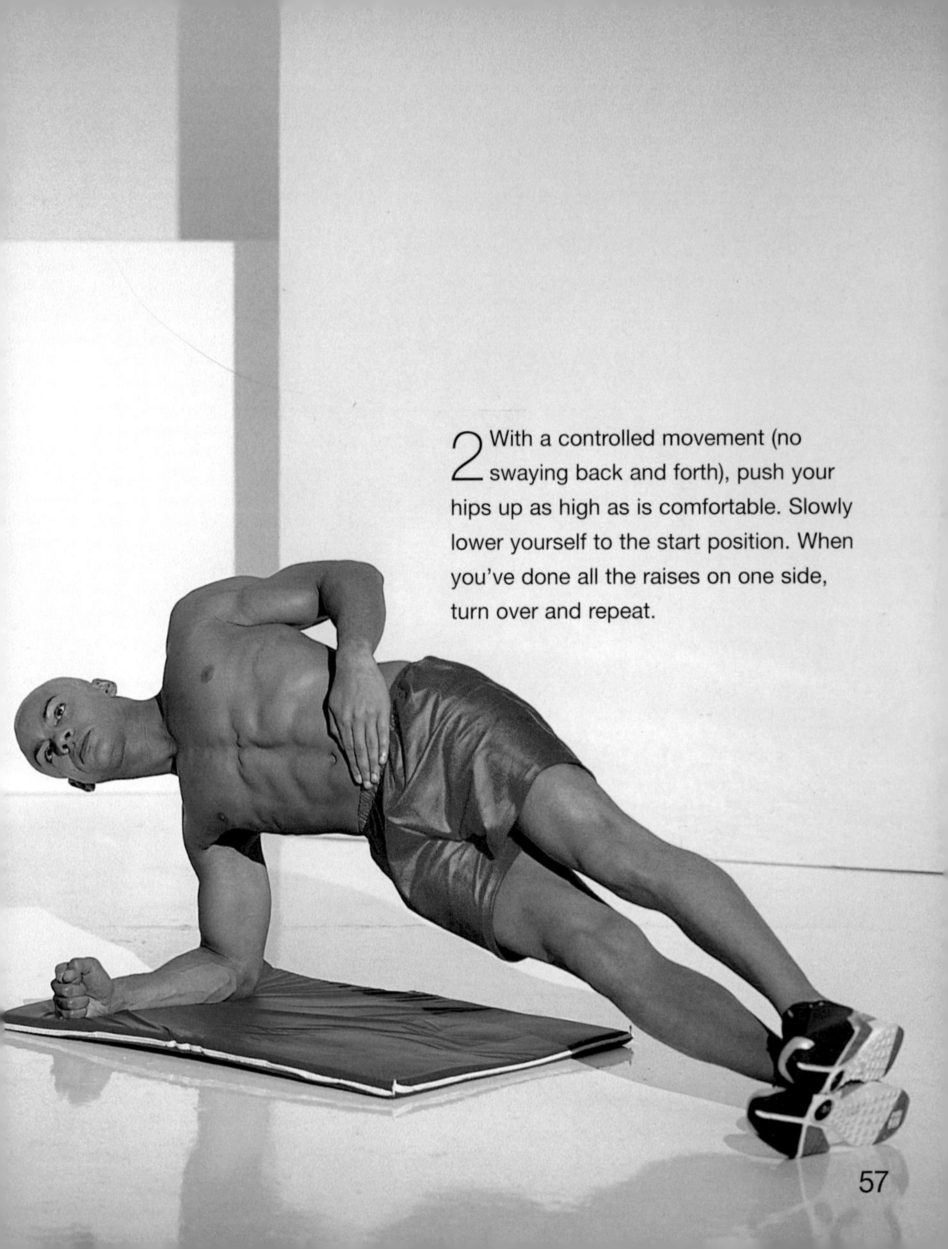

2 With a controlled movement (no swaying back and forth), push your hips up as high as is comfortable. Slowly lower yourself to the start position. When you've done all the raises on one side, turn over and repeat.

essential

stretches

To round off this workout, do the same stretches you did at the end of the first routine. Stretch your tightest or weakest side first. And take it slowly – this is time spent wisely.

1 hip flexor

Kneel on both knees, then step forwards with one foot. Keep your other knee on the floor. Rest your hands on the extended knee. Slide your back leg behind you. Feel the stretch in the front of your hip. Hold for 10–12 seconds. Repeat with your other leg.

2 cobra stretch

Lie on your front with your elbows tucked in close to your body. Keeping your hips on the floor, push your torso up until you're supporting your upper body on your elbows and forearms. Keep your neck relaxed. Hold for 15 seconds, then slowly return to the start position.

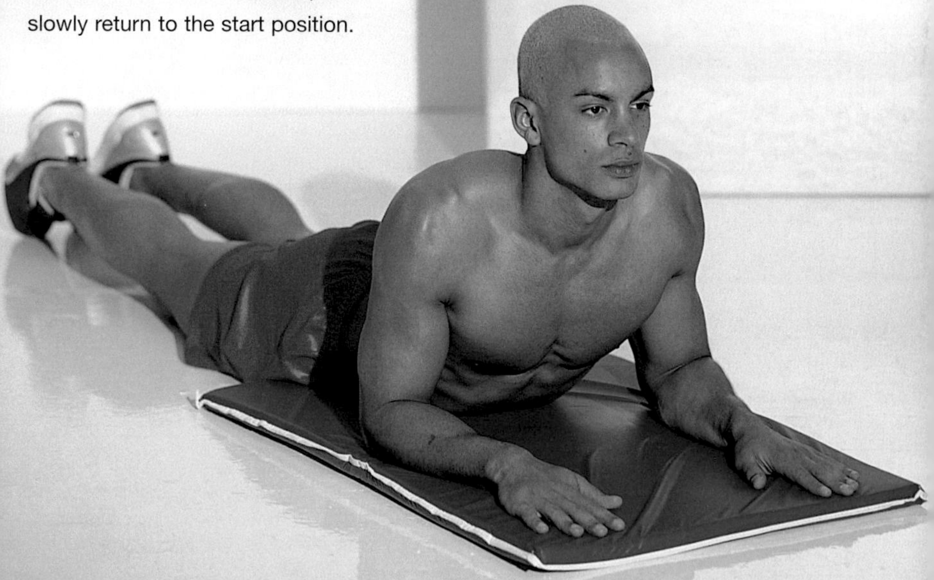

3 cat stretch

Position yourself on your hands and knees, with your back straight. Push your spine upwards to create a curve in the middle of your back. Hold for 5 seconds, then slowly return to the start position.

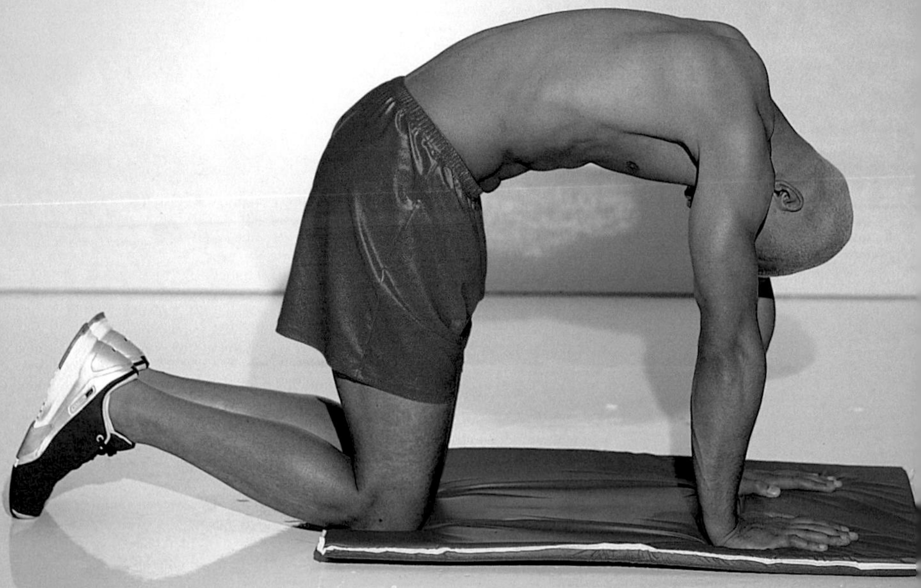

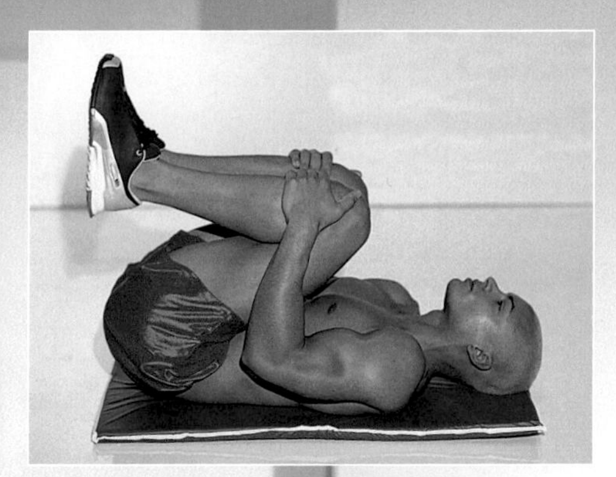

5 lower back stretch

Lie on your back, holding the tops of your shins with both hands. Gently pull your knees in close to your body until you can feel the stretch in your lower back. Hold for 10 seconds, then slowly return to the start position.

4 spine rotation

Lie on your back, with your arms stretched out at shoulder level. Bend both legs to 90°, then drop your knees to the side so one knee is touching the floor. Keep your shoulder blades flat on the floor, but don't force the stretch. Hold for 15 seconds, then slowly return to the start position. Repeat on your other side.

Q&A

fuel injection

I see other guys going into the gym with bottles of water. Should I be doing the same?

Most definitely. In fact, you shouldn't even think about setting foot inside the gym without a bottle that holds at least a litre (1¾ pints). It doesn't matter too much what kind of water it is (tap water is fine), but steer well clear of the carbonated stuff. Workouts are pretty sweaty affairs and drinking water during the session tops up your body's fluid levels. So much is obvious perhaps. But there's another reason for taking water in with you: exercise depletes large amounts of it from your muscles, and a process called acidic build-up can then set in. It's this that's responsible for any stiffness and soreness in your muscles. So, if only to avoid that day-after feeling, keep yourself well-hydrated during your workouts.

My diet's already fairly healthy. Do I need to cut out fat altogether?

Probably not, though it generally pays to monitor what you eat. Limit your intake of saturated fats (the ones that are solid at room temperature), but keep your consumption of healthy omega-3 oils (the sort you find in salmon and mackerel) high. If your weight's okay, never be tempted to cut too many calories, by the way – you'll simply end up burning muscle tissue. Stay in tune with your body and tinker with the number of calories you have from week to week if need be.

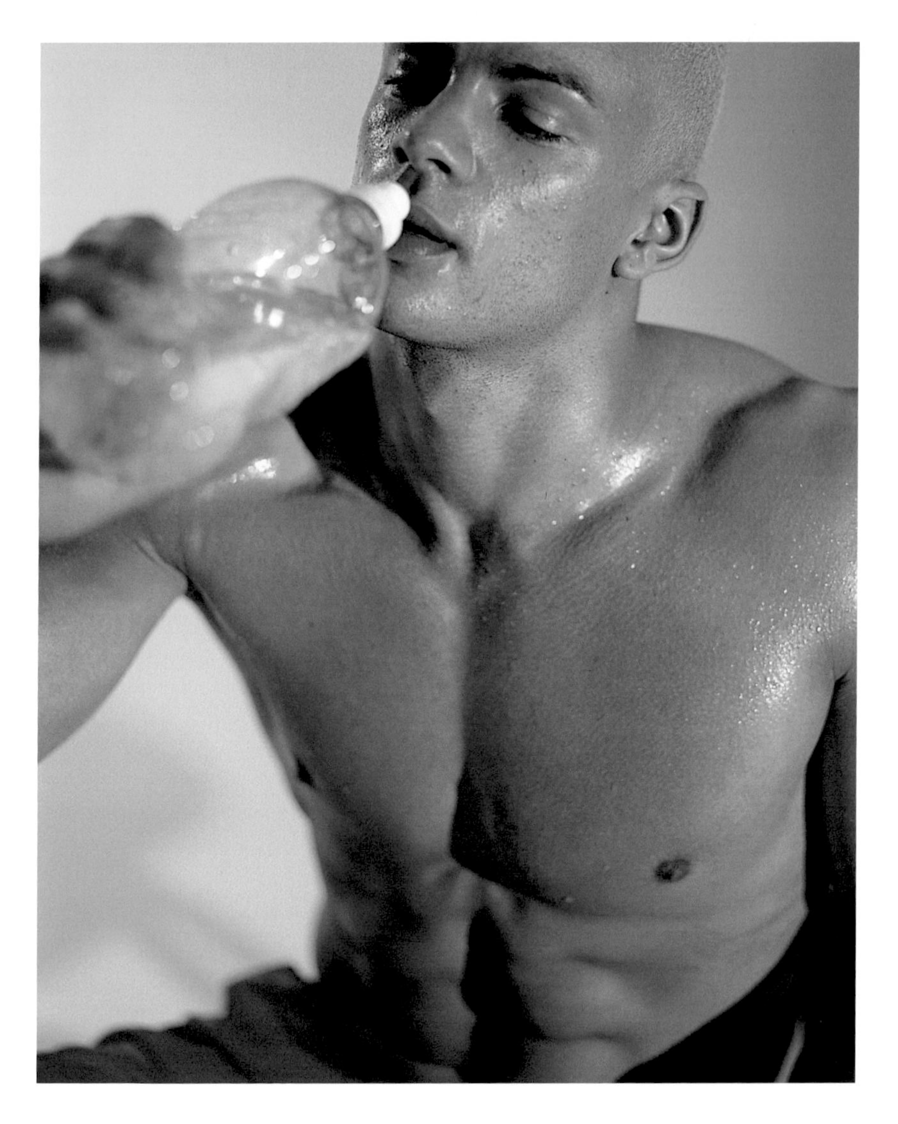

workout three

Aka ‘the fitness ball routine’. To reach those hard-to-get-at muscles in the deeper parts of your abdomen, here’s a workout I designed around the fitness ball. Abs work has never been such a blast…

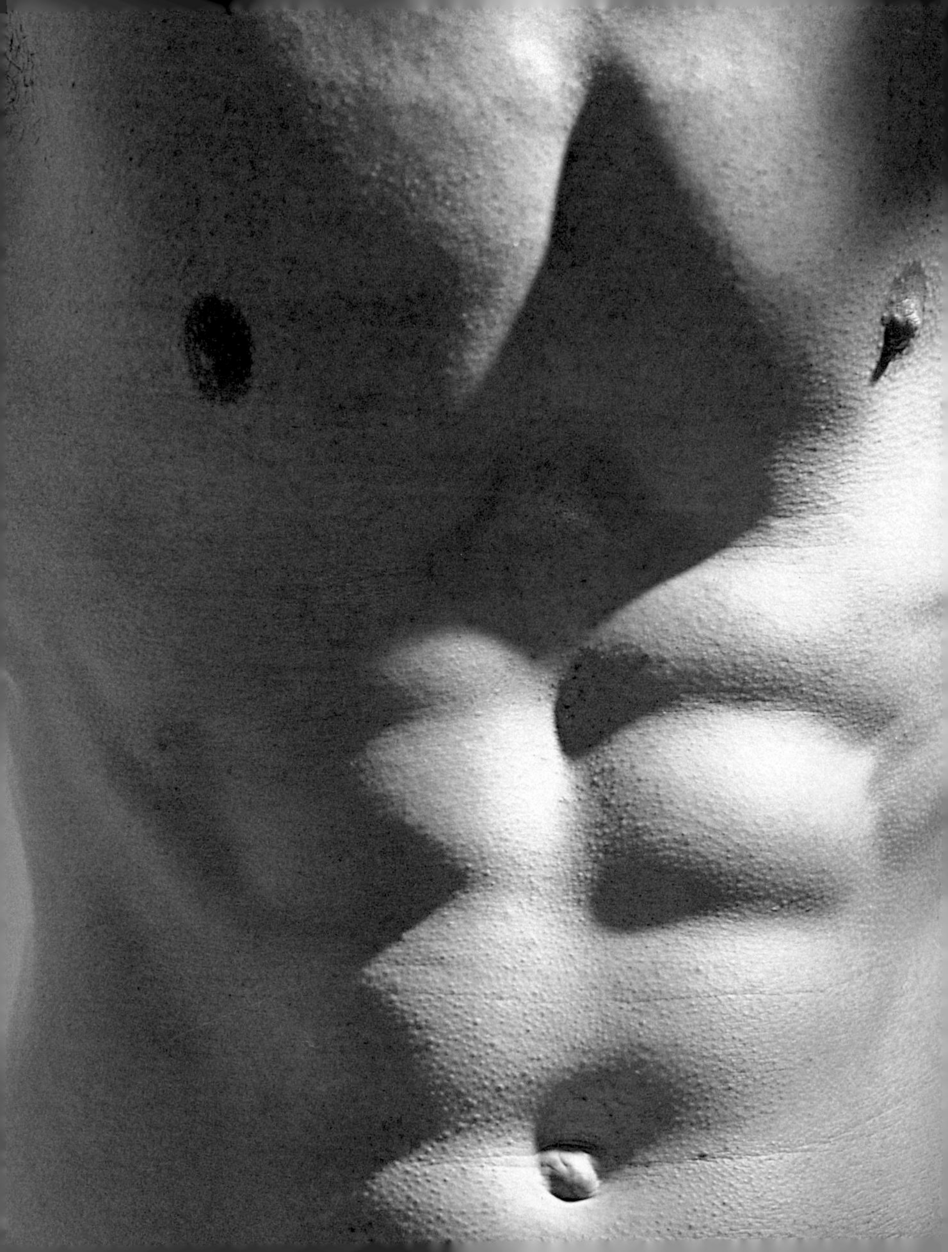

warm-up

Get yourself physically and psychologically geared up for the workout once again by warming up on the rower or cross-trainer for 5–10 minutes. This time is vital despite the fact that you're working only a small area like your abs.

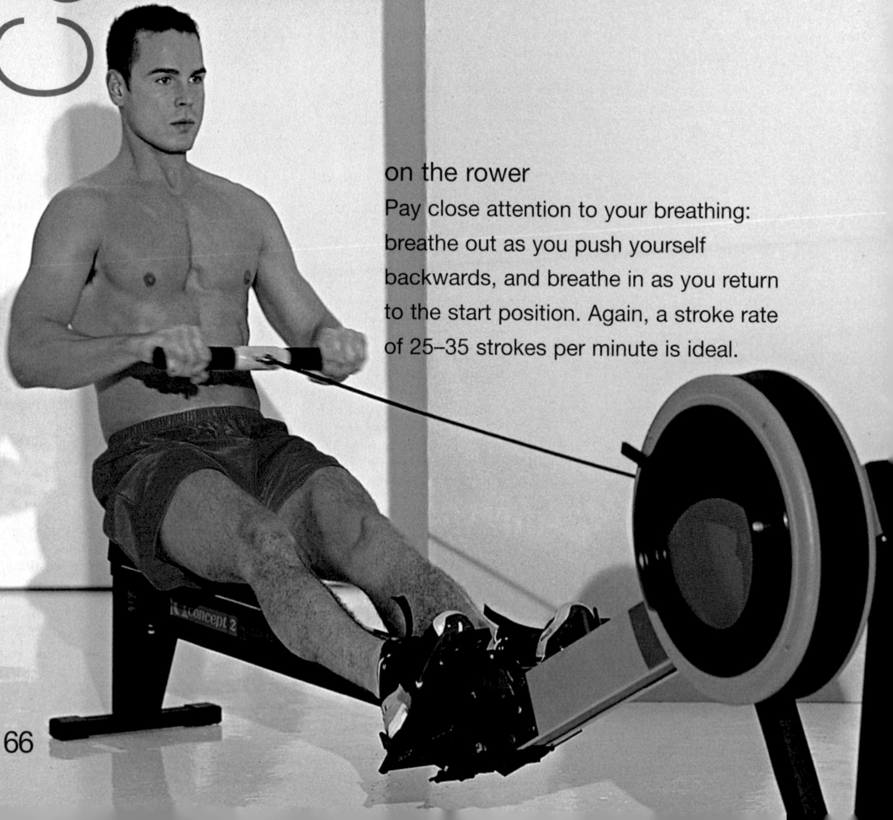

on the rower

Pay close attention to your breathing: breathe out as you push yourself backwards, and breathe in as you return to the start position. Again, a stroke rate of 25–35 strokes per minute is ideal.

on the cross-trainer

Make sure you work your arms as hard as your legs. It's easy to let them coast. Again, a stroke rate of 120–140 strokes per minute is ideal.

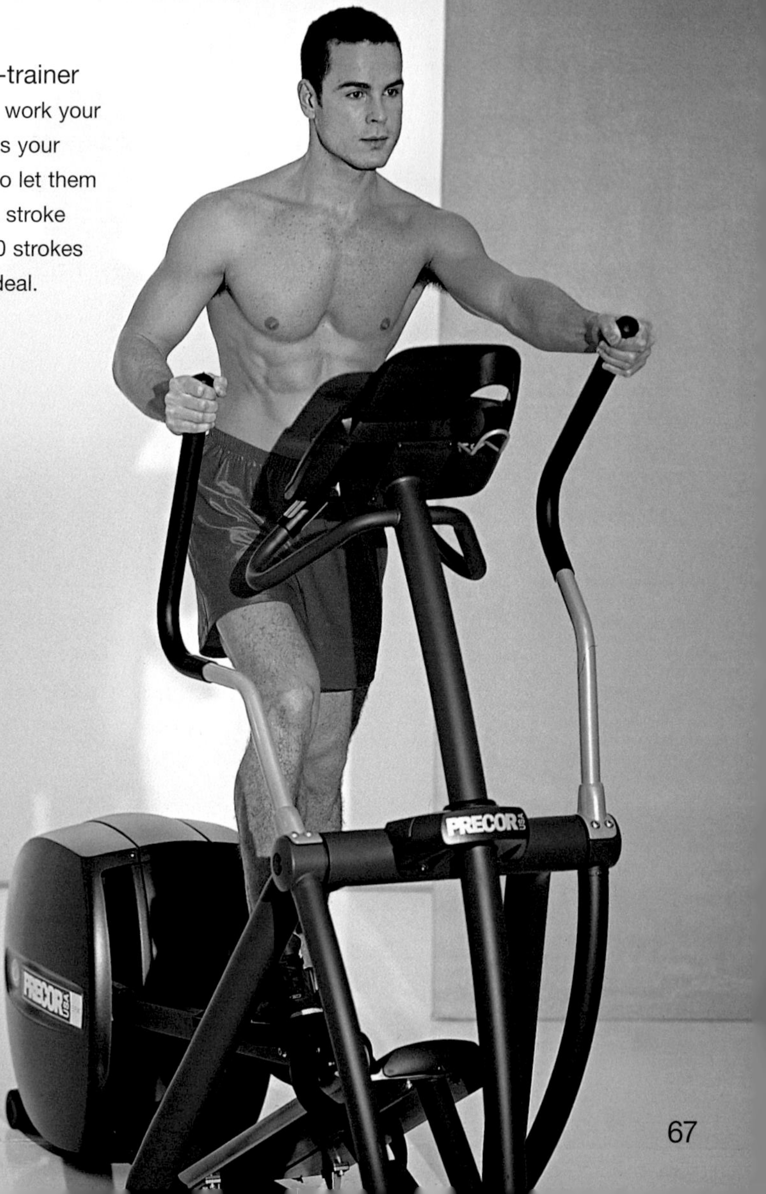

ball

sit-up

I like this exercise because it's simple but very effective: lying on the ball makes you work your lower abs harder and increases the stretch on your back.

level ① do 20 reps

level ② do 30 reps

1 Lie with the ball positioned securely between your buttocks and the bottom of your shoulder blades. Plant your feet on the floor about hip-width apart in front of you. Keep your hips in a neutral position (don't tilt your pelvis backwards). Place your hands by your ears.

2 Crunch your abs and bring your chest and shoulders forwards towards your hips. Keep your pelvis still and relaxed. Slowly return to the start position.

do it right

fitness balls

Fitness balls (sometimes called Swiss balls or stability balls) are a popular piece of equipment in most gyms. They're primarily used for abs work, but are great as an alternative 'bench' for free-weight work. In the correct hands, they can increase the intensity of most exercises.

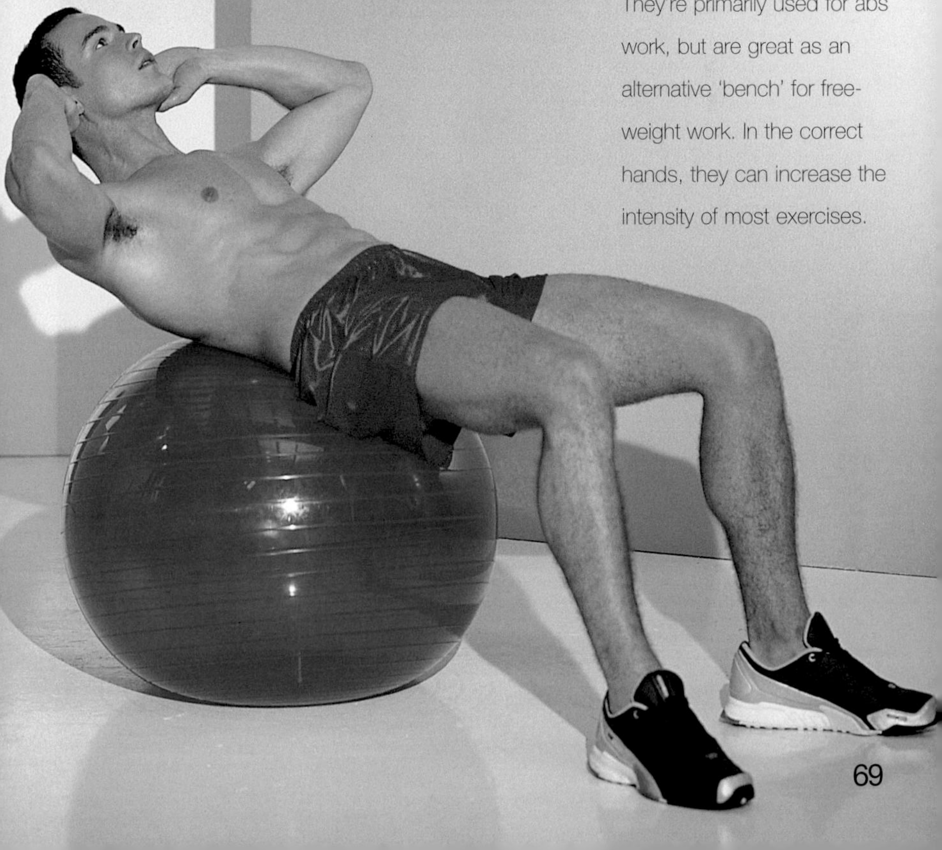

ball

oblique

The position you adopt for this exercise is unique. It allows you to work your abs and obliques dynamically.

level ① do 15 reps per side

level ② do 25 reps per side

1 Lie sideways on the ball with the ball positioned securely between your hips and your armpit. Place one foot behind the other at the base of a wall. Place your hands by your ears, elbows out to the side. Keep your head and neck in line with your spine.

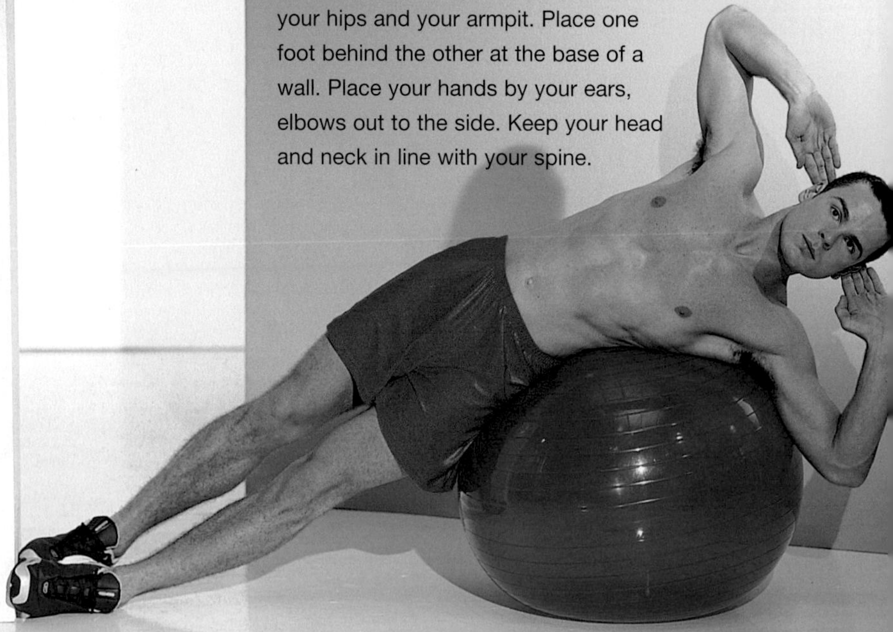

2 Using your obliques, pull your upper body up sideways in a straight line. Keep your neck in line with your spine. Slowly return to the start position. When you've done all the obliques on one side, turn over and repeat.

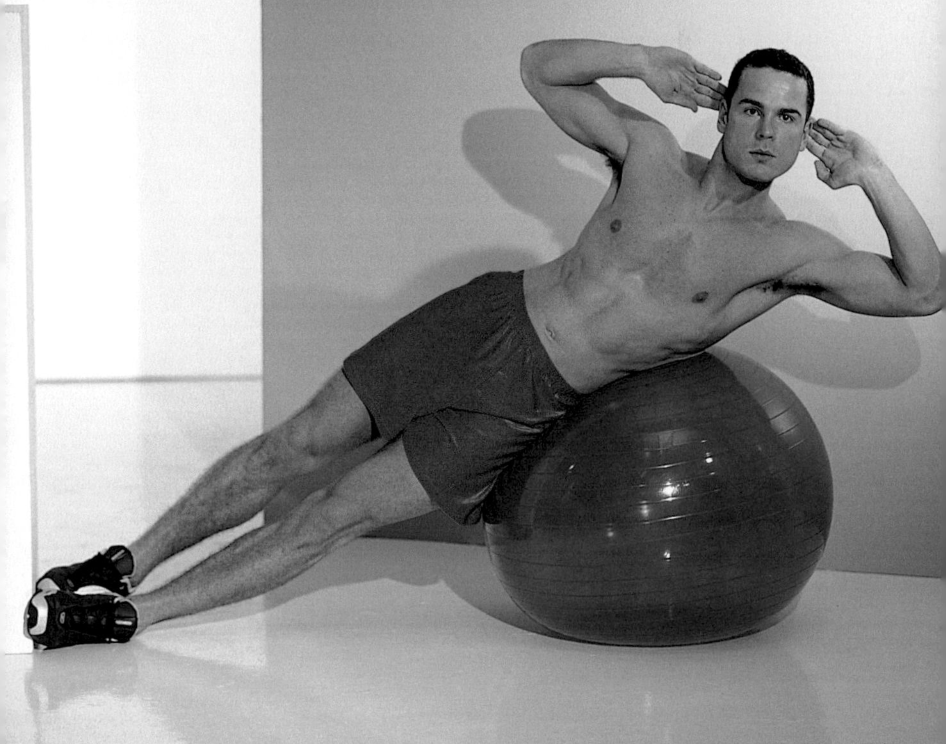

supported crunch

Supporting your lower legs on the fitness ball tilts your pelvis towards you. This limits the amount of space you can work in and makes the exercise more difficult. Make sure you keep the ball still and your legs relaxed.

level ① do 20 reps

level ② do 40 reps

1 Lie on your back with your knees bent at about 90° and your feet together on top of the ball. Place your hands by your ears, elbows out to the sides.

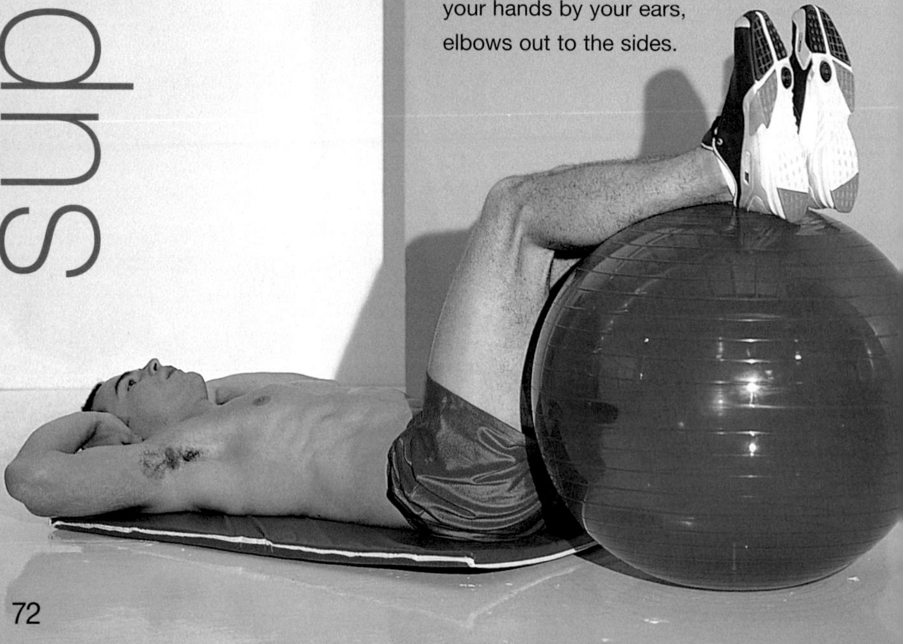

2 Tighten your abs and raise your shoulders off the floor, keeping your head in line with your spine. Slowly return to the start position.

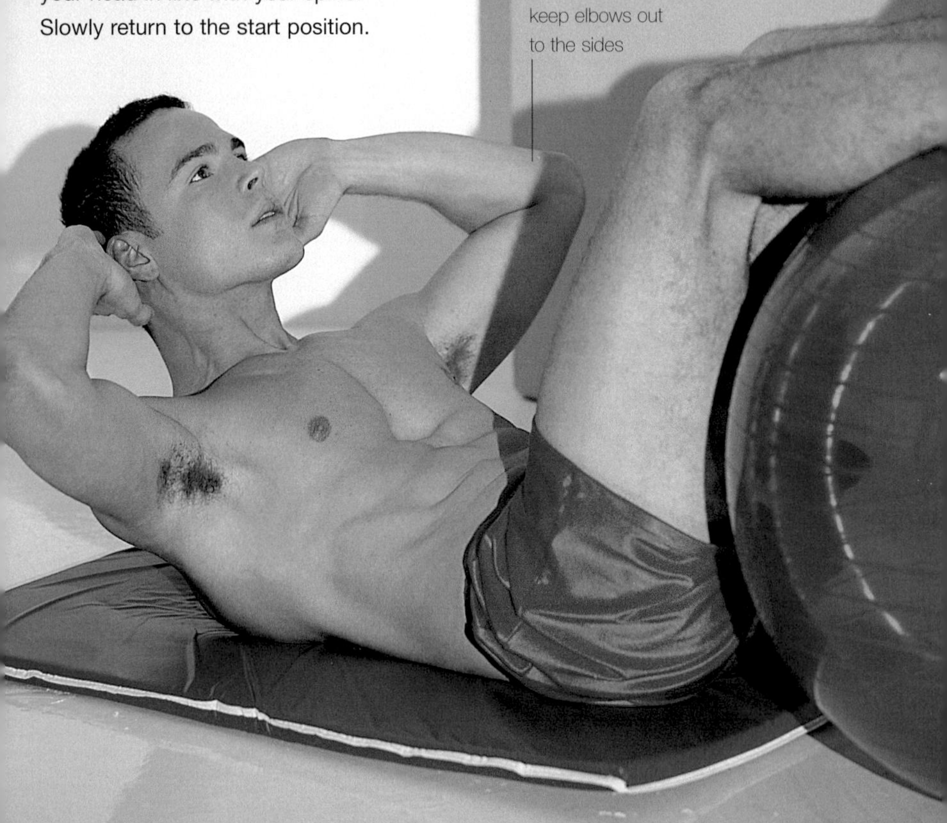

keep elbows out to the sides

supported oblique crunch

Here, you're lifting and rotating rather than simply pivoting on one shoulder. The lift works your abs and the rotation tests your obliques.

level ① do 15 reps per side

level ② do 30 reps per side

1 Lie on your back with your knees bent at about 90° and your feet together on top of the ball. Place your hands by your ears, elbows out to the sides.

2 Tighten your abs and curl one shoulder and elbow up towards your opposite knee. Slowly return to the start position. When you've done all the crunches on one side, switch to your other side and repeat.

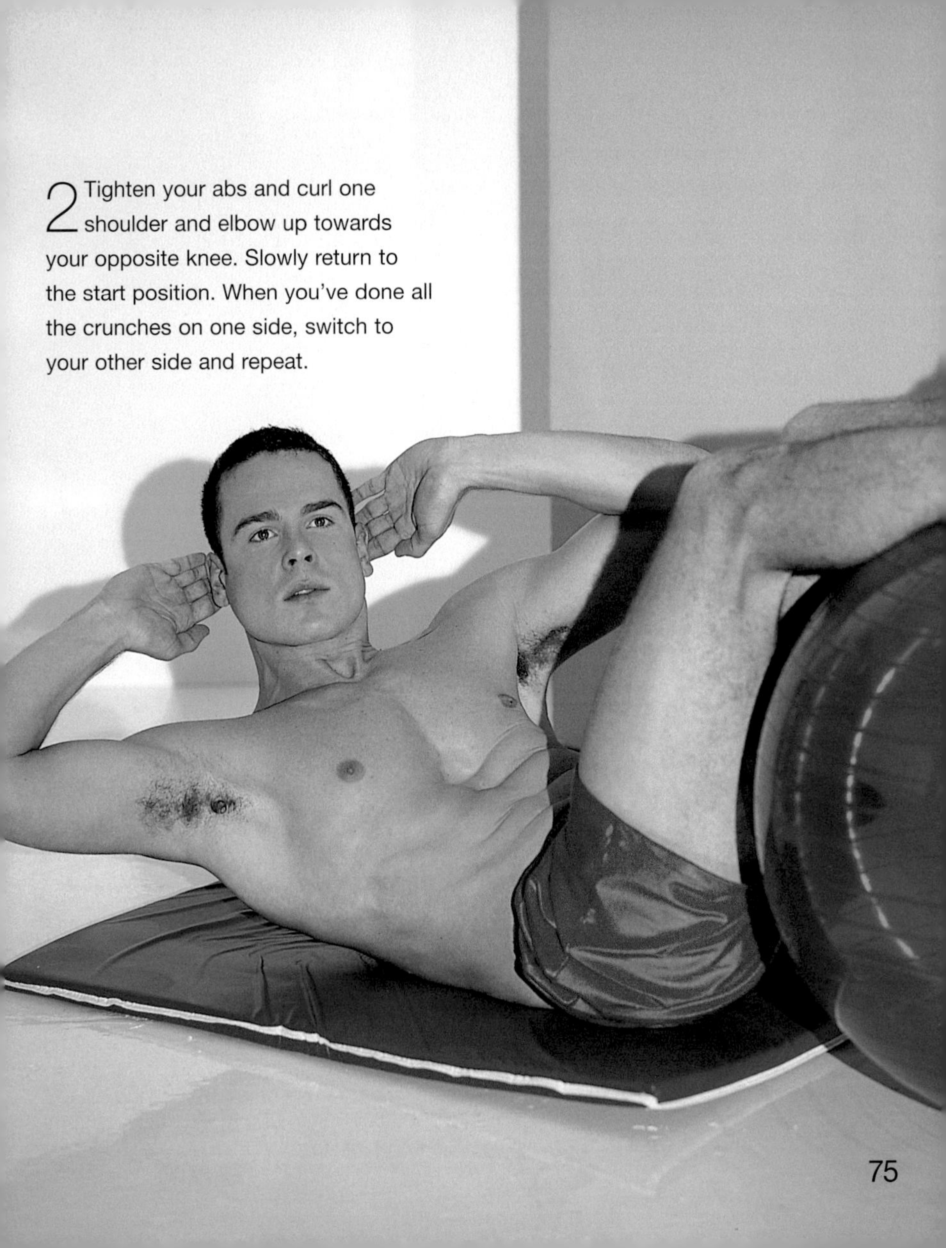

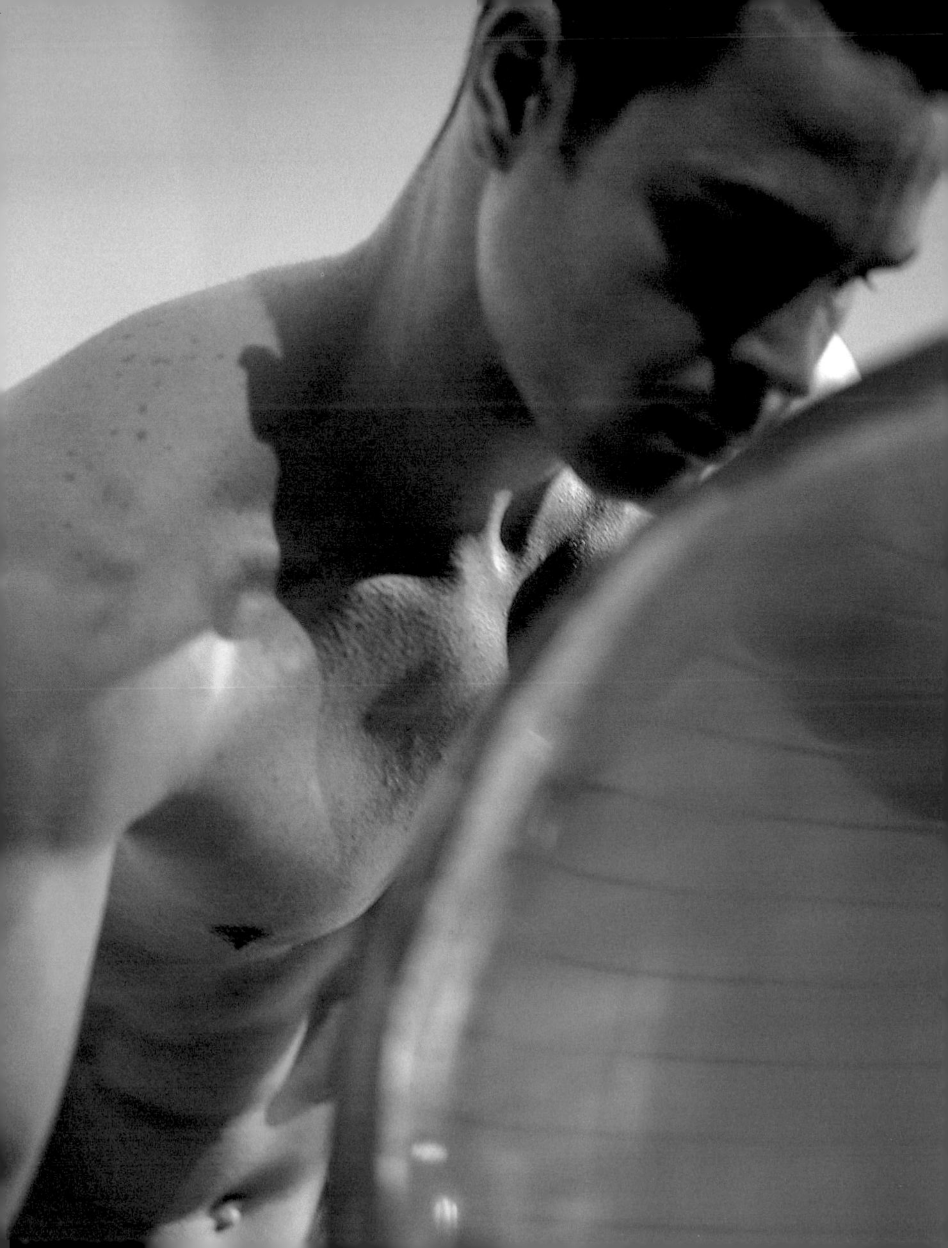

Take the exercises gently: don't just go hell for leather. Check constantly that you're maintaining control in your abs (rather than relying on the momentum of your body). And remember: a few high-quality reps are better than many low-quality ones.

ball

pike

This looks good and works better. Your arms need to be pretty strong, but it's your abs that are doing most of the work (provided you keep your legs straight). Practise it, then challenge your mates to have a go.

level ① do 15 reps

level ② do 25 reps

1 With feet together, rest your shins on the ball. Support your upper body by placing your hands just over shoulder-width apart directly under your shoulders. Keep a straight line from your head to your toes.

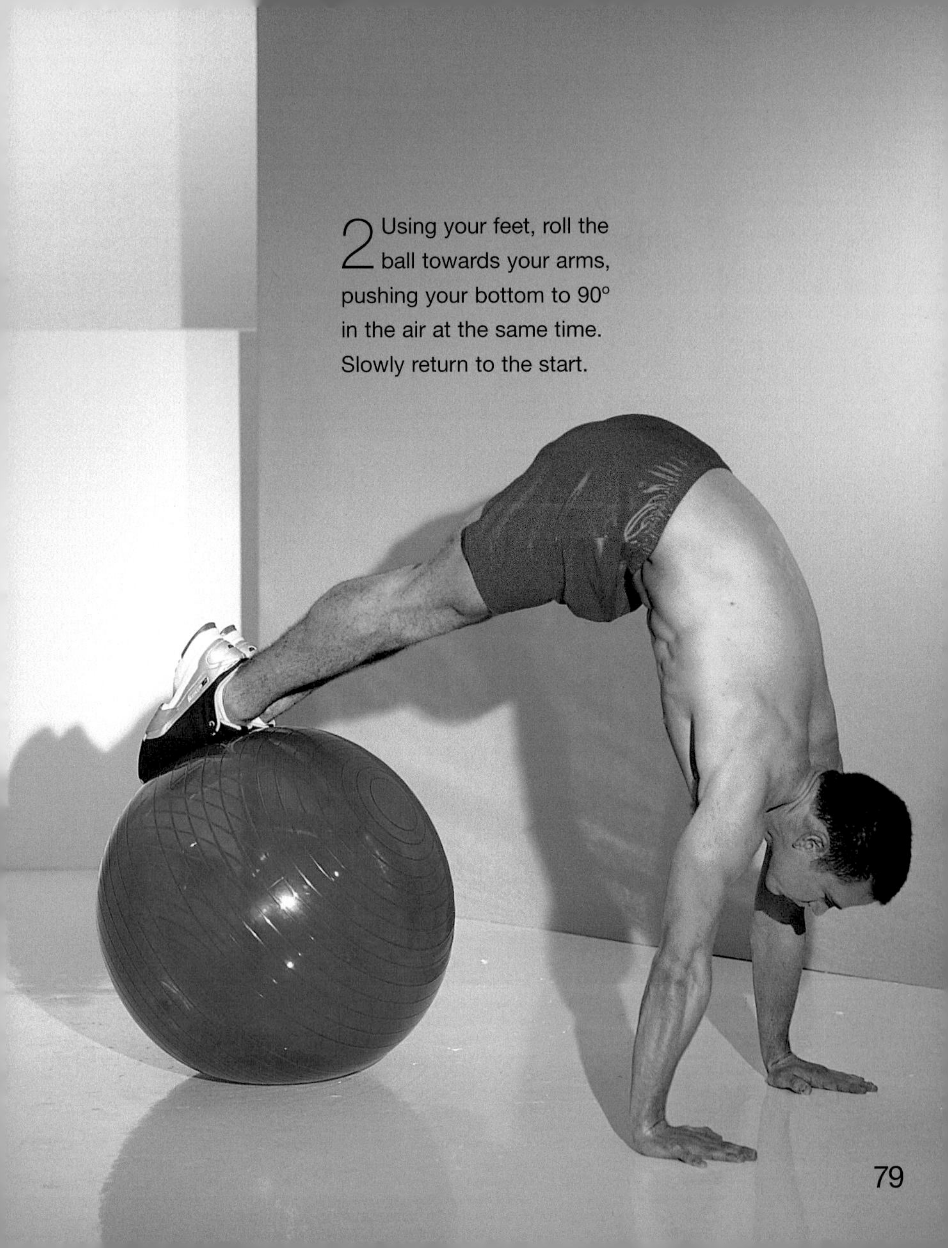

2 Using your feet, roll the ball towards your arms, pushing your bottom to 90° in the air at the same time. Slowly return to the start.

ball

bridge

This is a great test of your abs and your 'synergistic' muscles (the groups of muscles you're using here to keep your balance). Once you get better at it, move the ball from the shin position towards your toes. It makes it trickier still.

level ① hold for 30 secs

level ② hold for 60 secs

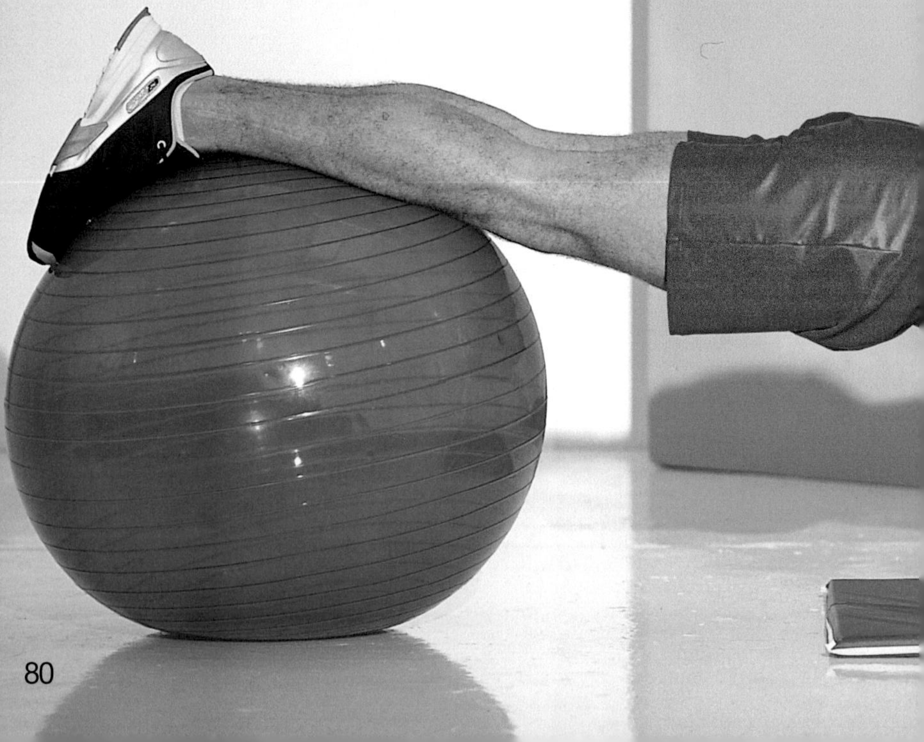

Rest your shins on the ball, keeping your feet together. Support your upper body by placing your elbows and forearms directly below your shoulders. Maintain the position with your abs, taking care to keep a straight line from your ankles to your shoulders.

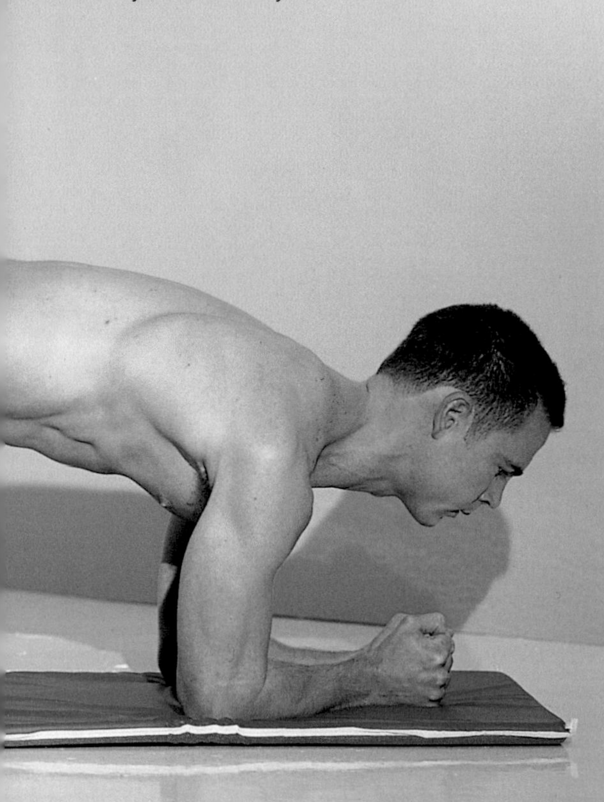

eat lean

when to eat

I've designed these workouts to strengthen and define your stomach muscles, but for a perfect six-pack, you also need to watch when you eat.

- Make sure you have a substantial breakfast every day. In an ideal world, you'll eat enough to last you right through to lunchtime.
- Graze throughout the day rather than eating two or three blow-out meals. 'Strategic snacking' keeps your body satisfied and avoids those energy dips that tempt you to reach for quick-fix foods.
- Eat your last meal of the day at least 2 hours before you go to bed. And keep it light.

reverse curl with ball

It might look odd and feel odd, but this ball pick-up will work your stomach muscles hard. Focus on using your abs and keeping your arms relaxed.

level ① do 20 reps

level ② do 40 reps

1 Lie on your back with your arms by your sides. Rest your heels and calves about knee-width apart on the ball.

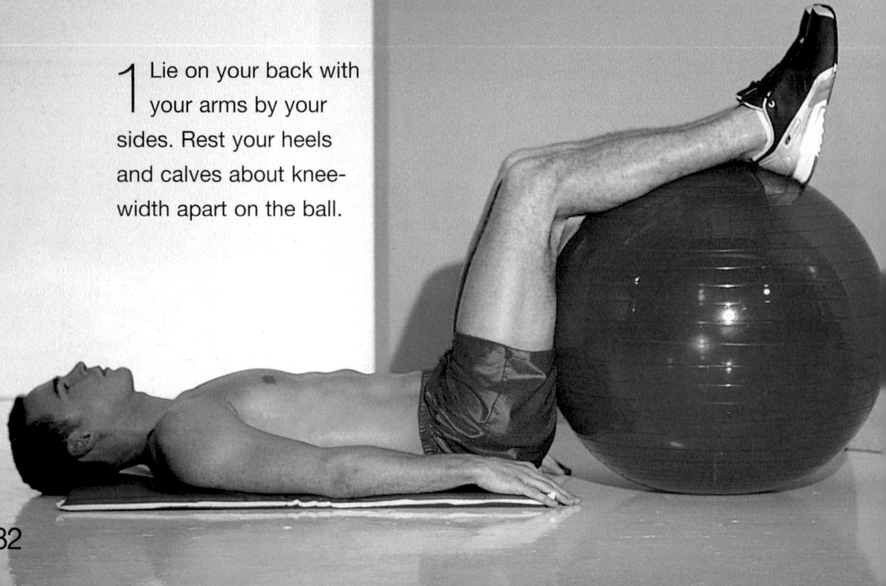

2 Tense your abs and, holding the ball between your heels and your thighs, raise it off the floor. Gripping the ball tightly, bring your thighs towards you until your lower back is just about to leave the floor. Slowly return to the start.

eat lean

no-no foods

If you're serious about your six-pack, these are the foods you should avoid: anything oily, starchy, or heavy, processed foods, red meat, dairy products, biscuits, cakes, and chocolate.

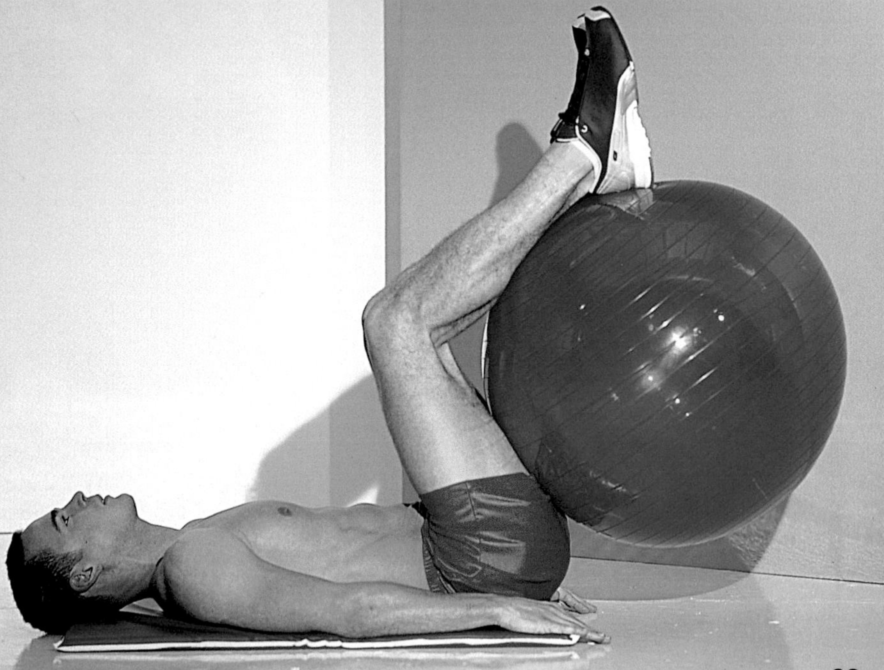

essential stretches

Finish up once again with the stretch moves. If you have time, perform each one two or three times – the more you stretch the more you benefit.

1 hip flexor

Kneel on both knees, then step forwards with one foot. Keep your other knee on the floor. Rest your hands on the extended knee. Slide your back leg out behind you. Feel the stretch in the front of your hip. Hold for 10–12 seconds. Repeat with your other leg.

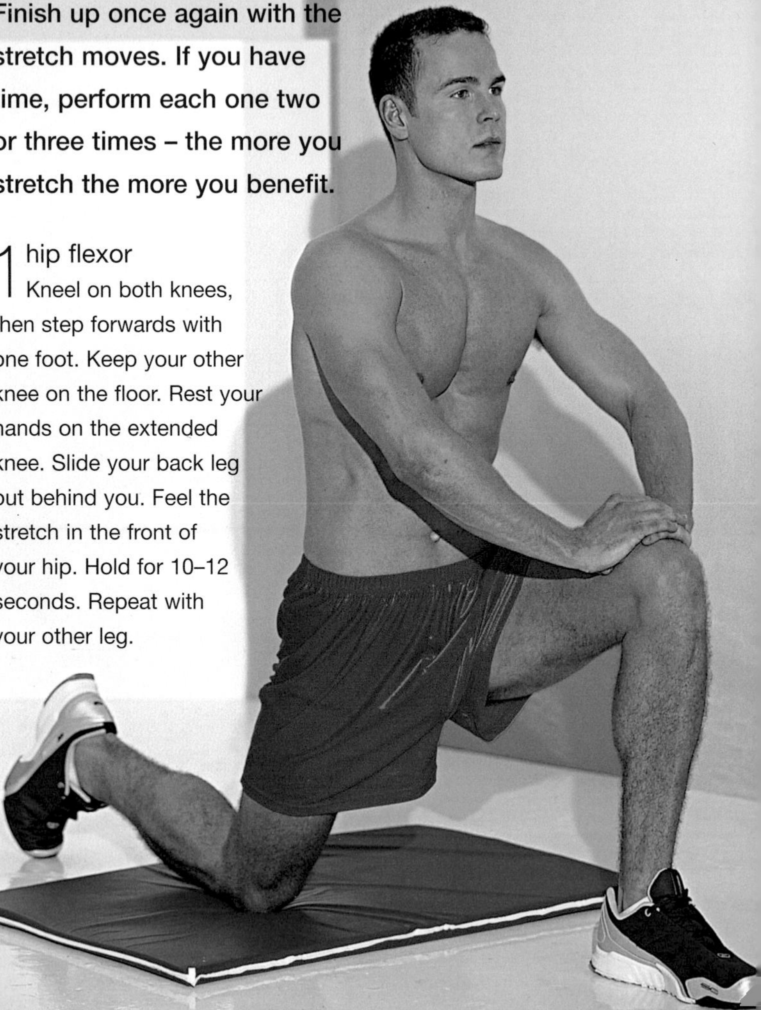

2 cobra stretch

Lie on your front with your elbows tucked in close to your body. Keeping your hips on the floor, push your torso up until you're supporting your upper body on your elbows and forearms. Keep your neck relaxed. Hold for 15 seconds, then slowly return to the start position.

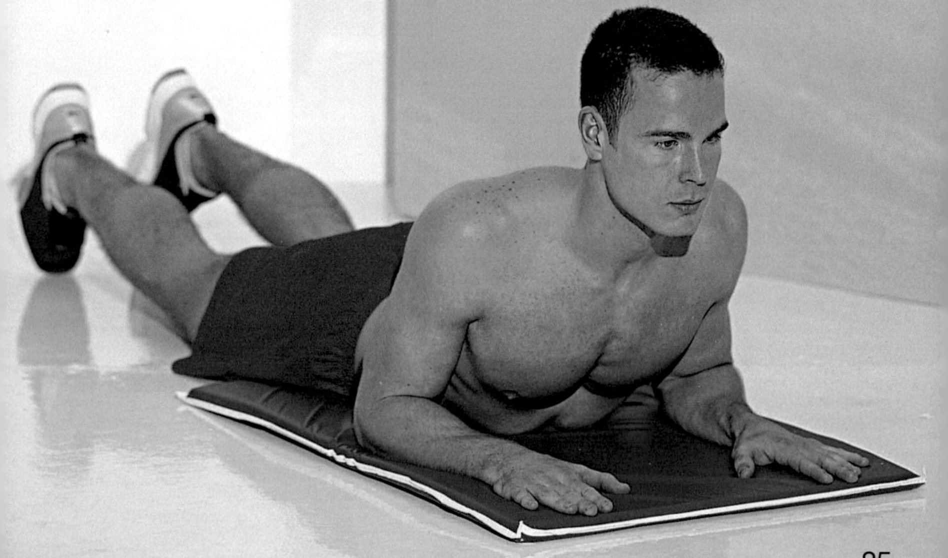

3 cat stretch

Position yourself on your hands and knees, with your back straight. Push your spine upwards to create a curve in the middle of your back. Hold for 5 seconds, then slowly return to the start position.

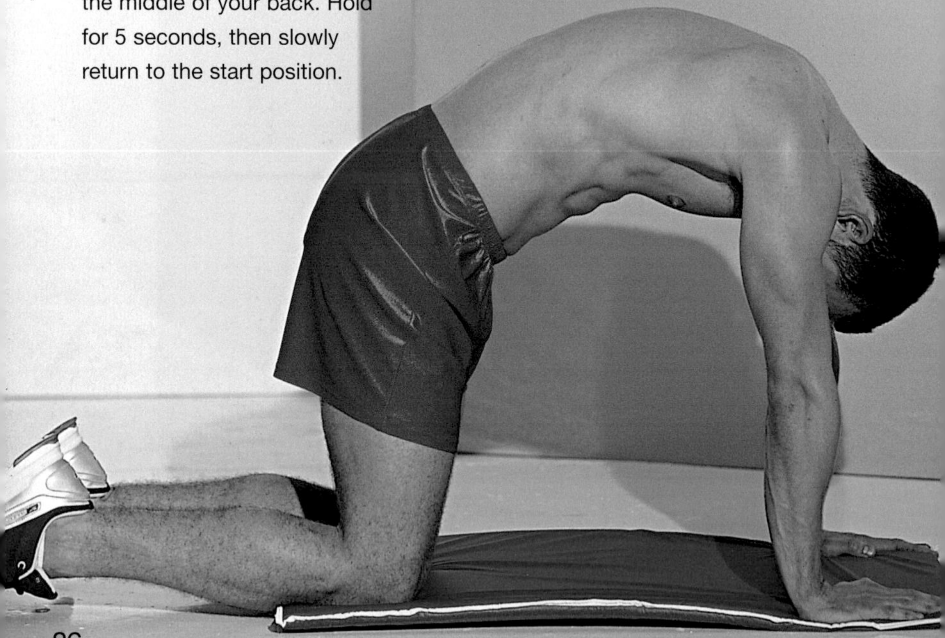

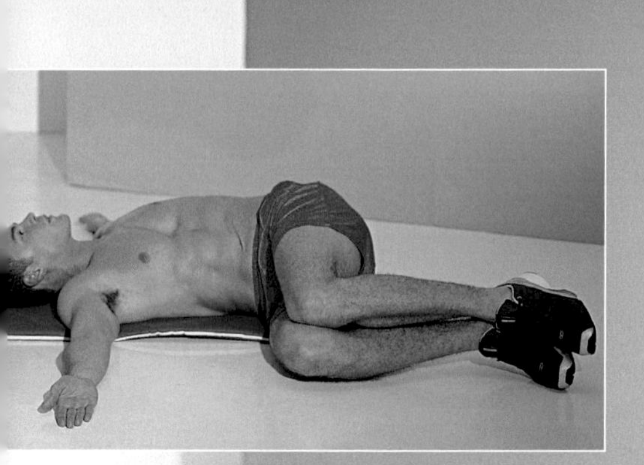

4 spine rotation

Lie on your back, with your arms out at shoulder level. Bend both legs to 90° and drop your knees to the side so one knee is touching the floor. Keep your shoulder blades flat on the floor, but don't force the stretch. Hold for 15 seconds. Return to the start. Repeat on your other side.

5 lower back stretch

Lie on your back, holding the tops of your shins with both hands. Gently pull your knees in close to your body until you can feel the stretch in your lower back. Hold for 10 seconds, then slowly return to the start position.

Q&A

staying toned

Now I've got my six-pack, how do I hang on to it?

The answer is – of course – to keep on exercising. From time to time, it's also worth checking that you're performing the exercises correctly – sloppy work makes for a sloppy body. Make sure, for instance, that you're maintaining control in the abdominal area rather than using the momentum of your body to do the required number of reps. And take it slowly – you'll derive far more benefit from a few high-quality reps than from many low-quality ones.

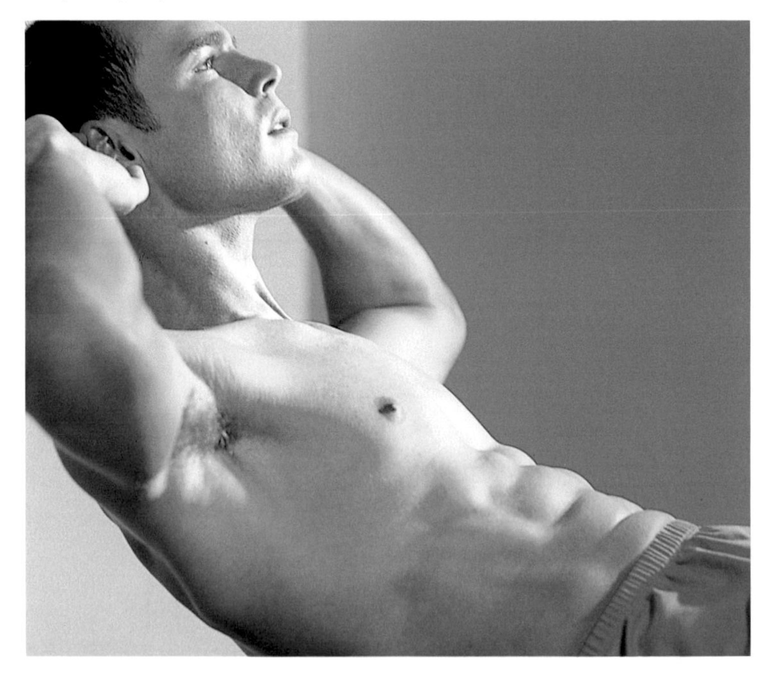

I want to stay looking ripped. How often do I need to work out from now on?

At the beginning of the book, I recommended you aim to work out every other day. This is fine for the first six weeks or so, but after that I think you can safely reduce the number of sessions to five or six a fortnight. If you're looking to burn body fat, you might want to alternate them with sessions that are pure cardio work. With time on your hands, of course, you can carry on working out every other day, but never be tempted to overtrain. While it's true that abs seem to recover a little more quickly than many other muscle groups, they still need rest. Stick to my rule of thumb of allowing at least 48 hours between ab workouts. And consider increasing the intensity you exercise at (*see below*).

What should I do when the workouts in this book start to seem a bit easy?

Resist giving yourself a pat on the back and step up the work by changing your exercise level instead. If you've been working at level ①, upgrade yourself to level ② and start the workouts afresh. If you're already on level ②, do the workouts as usual, but once you get to the last exercise, go back to the beginning and do them all again. Overleaf you'll also find some variations on the basic sit-up. I made these more difficult by altering the position of your arms or by adding a medicine ball or exertube – principles you can apply to some of the other exercises in the book.

Q&A

making it harder

I find the sit-up quite simple now. Are there more difficult versions I can move on to?

Yes, there are. Like many other exercises for your abs, you can increase the difficulty by altering the position of your arms or by incorporating a prop such as a medicine ball or exertube. Here are three variations.

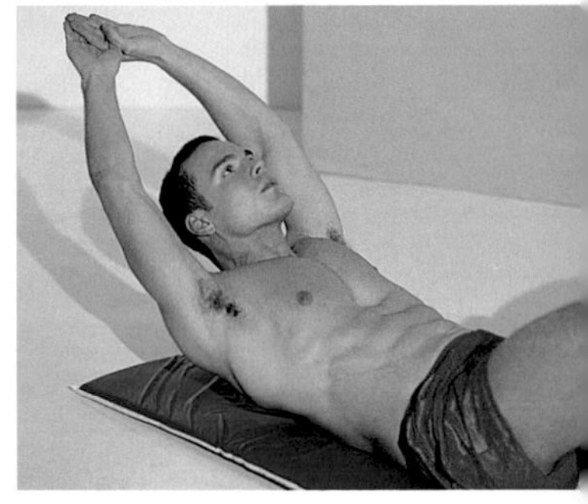

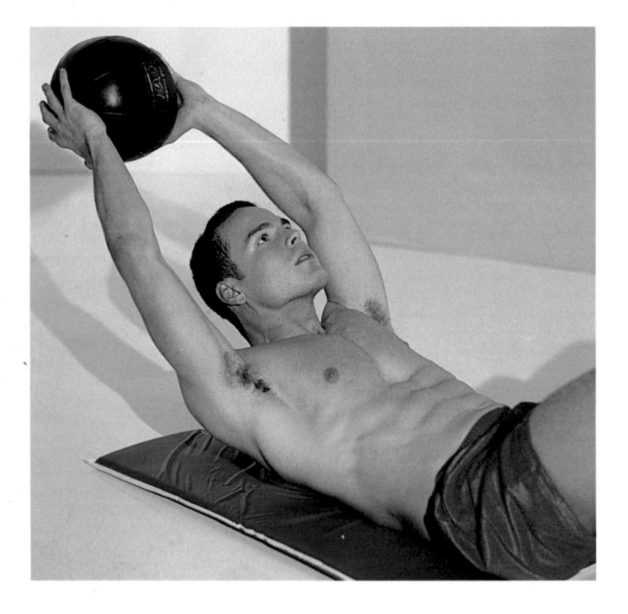

Above For a slightly more difficult version of the sit-up, try doing it with hands extended behind your head.

Left Once extending your arms behind your head no longer poses a challenge, incorporate a medicine ball, holding it in the same position.

And when you want to make the sit-up really demanding, secure an exertube around a pole or post behind you. Adjust it so that it offers plenty of resistance.

For more information about exertubes, see pages 92–93

useful information

which fitness level?

Before you start the workouts, you need to know your fitness level – ① or ②. If you're currently taking little or no exercise, start at level ①. If you already do 30 minutes or more cardio exercise (that's enough to make you puff and sweat) once a week or more, start at level ②. If the exercises start to seem a bit easy and you're working at level ①, upgrade yourself to level ②. If you're already working at level ②, do the workout as usual, but when you get to the last exercise, go back to the beginning and do them all again.

how often to perform the workouts

Aim to perform each workout at least once a week. Do them alternately. Never repeat the same workout within a 48-hour period – like any other muscles in your body, your abs need a rest. It's fine to do some other form of training on this day off, though.

working out at home

If you invest in a fitness ball, you could well do these routines at home. Remember to warm up first, though. Go for a short run, or cycle or swim.

a word about fitness balls and exertubes

You'll sometimes see fitness balls called Swiss balls, stability balls, gym balls, and back balls. I think they're great: they improve your balance as well as toning your muscles. They come in three sizes according to your height and weight. They're available from most sports shops and department stores, but in case you have problems I've given you some suppliers below.

If you were unfamiliar with exertubes before, you'll have seen them in the sit-up variations on pages 90–91. They're another great piece of kit – they're cheap, easy to use, and light enough to carry around with you. They come in colour-coded strengths, ranging from low-resistance to high.

suppliers of fitness balls and exertubes

If you have problems finding fitness balls and exertubes in your local shops, you can order them from the following suppliers:

In the UK
Physique Management
0870 60 70 381
www.physique.co.uk

In Australia
www.simplefitnesssolutions.com

In New Zealand
www.fitnessworks.co.nz

index

credits

author's credits

Thanks to everybody (too many of you to name, alas) who helped me with this book. A special thank you to the DK team, to Michael, Tracy, and Anna, in particular; to Russell for the great shots; to my own team, especially Nik, Richard, Jason, Ayo, and Alan; and to my brother Jon, who, as always, shared the workload with me.

For more information about Matt Roberts Personal Training, please contact:

matt roberts personal training
32–34 Jermyn St
London SW1Y 6HS
Tel: 020 7439 8800
www.personaltrainer.uk.com

publisher's credits

Thanks to our models Jon Firth and Lee Stafford from ModelPlan, and to Nessie at ModelPlan; to Matt's team of trainers Nik Cook, George Dick, Jason Hughes, Ayo Williams, and Alan Foley; to Toko at Hers for hair and make-up; to stylist Jo Atkins-Hughes; to photography assistant Nina Duncan; and to designer Janis Utton for her timely help. Many thanks to Reebok for the kind loan of trainers for this book (all enquiries 0800 30 50 50).

about the author

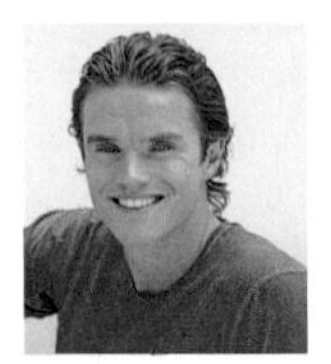

Matt Roberts, the UK's hottest personal trainer, began as an international sprinter. He went on to complete his studies at the American Council for Exercise and the American College of Sports Medicine. Affectionately known as 'the personal trainer to the stars', Matt has an enviable reputation for training celebrities, among them Sandra Bullock, Trudie Styler, Mel C, Natalie Imbruglia, Naomi Campbell, Tom Ford, John Galliano, and Faye Dunaway. Alongside this high-profile client list, Matt derives equal satisfaction from helping each of his clients meet their health and fitness goals. And in his quest to make fitness and good health accessible to everyone, he produces his own range of vitamins, home gym equipment, and body care products.